Workbook

Experiencing the World of the Counselor
A Workbook for Counselor Educators and Students

Edward Neukrug
Old Dominion University

Prepared by

Edward Neukrug
Old Dominion University

BROOKS/COLE
CENGAGE Learning

Australia • Brazil • Japan • Korea • Mexico • Singapore • Spain • United Kingdom • United States

© 2012 Brooks/Cole, Cengage Learning

ALL RIGHTS RESERVED. No part of this work covered by the copyright herein may be reproduced, transmitted, stored, or used in any form or by any means graphic, electronic, or mechanical, including but not limited to photocopying, recording, scanning, digitizing, taping, Web distribution, information networks, or information storage and retrieval systems, except as permitted under Section 107 or 108 of the 1976 United States Copyright Act, without the prior written permission of the publisher.

For product information and technology assistance, contact us at **Cengage Learning Customer & Sales Support, 1-800-354-9706**

For permission to use material from this text or product, submit all requests online at **www.cengage.com/permissions**
Further permissions questions can be emailed to **permissionrequest@cengage.com**

ISBN-13: 978-0-8400-3433-5
ISBN-10: 0-8400-3433-4

Brooks/Cole
20 Davis Drive
Belmont, CA 94002-3098
USA

Cengage Learning is a leading provider of customized learning solutions with office locations around the globe, including Singapore, the United Kingdom, Australia, Mexico, Brazil, and Japan. Locate your local office at: **www.cengage.com/global**

Cengage Learning products are represented in Canada by Nelson Education, Ltd.

To learn more about Brooks/Cole, visit **www.cengage.com/brookscole**

Purchase any of our products at your local college store or at our preferred online store **www.cengagebrain.com**

Printed in the United States of America
1 2 3 4 5 6 7 15 14 13 12 11

To My Wife Kristina and my Daughters Hannah and Emma:
The Experience of My Life

BRIEF CONTENTS

Introduction:..xiii

Chapter 1:	Counselor Identity: What, Who, and How?..	1
Chapter 2:	The Counseling Profession's Past, Present, and Future	13
Chapter 3:	Standards: Ethics, Accreditation, Credentialing, and Multicultural and Advocacy Competencies	23
Chapter 4:	Individual Approaches to Counseling...	31
Chapter 5:	Counseling Skills	47
Chapter 6:	Couples and Family Counseling	67
Chapter 7:	Group Work	77
Chapter 8:	Consultation and Supervision	86
Chapter 9:	Human Development: Normal and Abnormal	96
Chapter 10:	Career Development	109
Chapter 11:	Research and Evaluation	121
Chapter 12:	Testing and Assessment	131
Chapter 13:	Multicultural Counseling	142
Chapter 14:	Specialty Areas in Counseling	156
Chapter 15:	Going to Graduate School and Getting a Job	167

REFERENCES 173

APPENDICES
- A Perceptions of Ethical Conduct 179
- B Cross-Cultural Competencies and Objectives 182
- C Advocacy Competencies 186
- D Descriptions of Theoretical Orientations and Conceptual Orientations 189
- E Clinical Case Report 193
- F Consultation at a Mental Health Center 195
- G Understanding Your Holland Code 199
- H The Normal Curve 203
- I Numbers and Percentages of People and Religions in the World 204
- J The Graduate Degree Exploration Worksheet 206

TABLE OF CONTENTS

Introduction: vii

Chapter 1: Counselor Identity: What, Who, and How 1
Comparing Mental Health Professionals 1
Defining Guidance, Counseling, and Psychotherapy 1
Determining Characteristics of the Effective Counselor 1
Acquiring the Characteristics of the Effective Counselor 3
Assessing Self-Development 5
Am I ready to be a Counselor? A Self-Evaluation 6
Learning about Professional Associations 7
Advocating for Our Profession 9
Interviewing about Professionals in the Field 9
Conducting a Detailed Analysis of an Agency Where Counselors Work 10
Ethical, Legal, and Professional Vignettes 11

Chapter 2: The Counseling Profession's Past, Present, and Future 13
Important Names and Places 13
Are There Shamans Amongst Us? 15
What We Can Learn from Great People of History 16
Learning from Related Mental Health Professions 16
Historical Influences on Job Choice 16
A Look toward the Future 17
Are We Ready for Another "Paradigm Shift? 19
Keeping Yourself Well in a High Stress Occupation 19
Ethical, Legal, and Professional Vignettes 21

Chapter 3: Standards: Ethics, Accreditation, Credentialing, and Multicultural and Advocacy Competencies 23
Part I: Ethics 23
Developing Ethical Guidelines 23
Challenging Ethical Beliefs 23
Perceptions of Ethical Behaviors 23
Violating Ethics: The Consequences 24
Malpractice Insurance 24
Part II: Accreditation 24
Developing Accreditation Standards 24
Reviewing CACREP's Accreditation Standards 25
Accreditation of Related Professional Associations 25
Part III: Credentialing 25
Registration, Certification, and Licensing: What are the Differences? 25
Comparing Credentialing Processes 25
Part IV: Multicultural and Advocacy Competencies 27
Multicultural Counseling Competencies 27

Advocacy Competencies 28
Ethical, Legal, and Professional Vignettes 29

Chapter 4: Individual Approaches to Counseling 31
Your Theoretical Approach and Conceptual Orientation 31
Understanding Your View of Human Nature 36
Classification of Theoretical Approaches 37
Literature, Pop-Psychology, and Theory 38
Name that Theory 38
Differing Theoretical Orientations as Applied to Clients 39
The Implementation of Varying Theoretical Approaches 40
Using Cinema to Teach Counseling Theory 43
Adapting Theories to Brief and Solution-Focused Approaches 43
Disadvantages and Advantages of Brief Therapy and
    Solution-Focused Approaches 43
Eclecticism or Theoretical Integration 43
Ethical, Legal, and Professional Vignettes 45

Chapter 5: Counseling Skills 47
The Office Environment 47
Nonverbal Behavior and Touch 48
Listening Quiz 49
Hindrances to Effective Listening 49
Avoiding Counseling Clichés 50
Minimal Encourages (Words, Phrases, and or Gestures) 51
Making Empathic Responses 51
Advanced Empathy 54
Silence Is Golden 54
Basic Questions 54
Solution-Focused Questions 55
Self-Disclosure 56
Inadvertent and Intentional Modeling 56
Confrontation: Support and Challenge 57
Often Used Skills: Encouragement, Affirmations, Offering Alternatives,
    Information Giving, Advice Giving, Collaboration, Interpretation,
    and Respectful Curiosity 57
Assessing Counselor Skills 59
The Good versus the Bad Counselor 62
Writing Case Notes 62
Writing Case Reports 63
Ethical, Legal, and Professional Vignettes 63

Chapter 6: Couples and Family Counseling 67
General Systems Theory 67

Cybernetics 67
Applying an Understanding of Systems to Your Family 67
The Power of Langue in Family Development 68
Situational Stress in Families 69
Reflecting on Your Family of Origin 69
Family Development 69
Your Family Genogram 71
Working with a Family in Need 71
Comparing and Contrasting Family Therapy Approaches 71
Role Playing Family Therapy 73
Comparing Individual and Family Therapy Approache 73
Professional Associations 74
Ethical, Legal, and Professional Vignettes 75

Chapter 7: Group Work 77
Groups as a System 77
Wearing Labels 77
Advantages and Disadvantages of Groups 77
Ecological Concepts in Groups 78
Comparison of Groups: Free Association 78
Self-help Groups 78
Task Groups 79
Developing a Psychoeducational Group (Guidance Group) 79
Group Counseling 80
Group Therapy 80
Rules of Group Behavior 80
Comparison of Psychoeducational, Counseling, and Therapy Groups 81
Use of Theory in Group Work 81
Experiential Group Learning 83
Multicultural and Social Justice Issues in Group Work 83
Ethical, Legal, and Professional Vignettes 84

Chapter 8: Consultation and Supervision 86
Part I: Consultation 86
Examples of Consultation 86
Implementation of Different Types of Consultation 87
Consultation at a Mental Health Center 87
Consultation at a School 88
Consultation at a University 89
Utilizing Counseling Theory in Consultation 90
Part II: Supervision 91
Consultation and Supervision: Similarities and Differences 91
Supervision: A Systemic Process 91
Characteristics of the Effective Supervisor 91

Parallel Process 91
Styles of Supervision 91
Supervision of Graduate Students 94
Supervision in the Workplace 94
Ethical, Legal, and Professional Vignettes 94

Chapter 9: Human Development: Normal and Abnormal 96
Who Are You? 96
Reflecting on Your Personality Development 96
Defense Mechanisms 97
Examining Your Development 97
Comparison of Development Theories 101
Examining the Development of an Adult with a Developmental Disability ... 102
Counseling Gloria: A Developmental Perspective 103
Examining the Development of a Gifted Child 103
Counseling Joe: A Developmental Perspective 103
Developing Your Own Developmental Theory 104
Examining Differing Perspectives on Abnormal Behavior 104
Using the DSM 104
Classifying Medication in the Treatment of Emotional Problems 106
Ethical, Legal, and Professional Vignettes 107

Chapter 10: Career Development 109
Work, Avocations, Leisure Activities: What Are They? 109
Very Early Memories: Connecting Early Interests to Career Interests Today 109
Psychodynamic Factors and Career Choices 110
Personality Development and Career Choices 110
Situational Factors and Career Choices 110
Developmental Tasks and Career Choices 111
What Planet Do You Come From 112
Understanding Your Holland Code 114
Social Cognitive Career Theory 114
Constructivist Career Development 115
Integrating Career Development Theories 115
Understanding the Career Development of Others 117
Exploring Occupational Information 117
Assisting a Client (or Yourself) in Understanding Career Choices 118
Ethical, Legal, and Professional Vignettes 118

Chapter 11: Research and Evaluation 121
Understanding Paradigm Shifts 121
Conducting a Literature Search 121
Identifying Variables of Quantitative Research Studies 121
Developing Hypotheses and Research Questions 122

Steps You Might Use in Developing a Qualitative Studies 122
Critiquing a Journal Article 123
Designing a Research Study 123
Validating Qualitative Research 124
Threats to Internal Validity in Quantitative Research 124
Designing a Qualitative Study 125
Designing a Quantitative Study 126
Comparing Quantitative and Qualitative Research 126
Evaluating an Evaluation Form 126
Developing an Evaluation Form 127
Writing a Fictitious Manuscript Describing a Research Study or
    Program Evaluation 127
Comparing Different Kinds of Research and Evaluation 128
Ethical, Legal, and Professional Vignettes 128

Chapter 12: Testing and Assessment 131
Differences between Testing and Assessment 131
Sharing Experiences with Testing 131
Advantages and Disadvantages to Testing and Assessment 131
Types of Tests 131
Categories of Tests 132
Using Tests with Clients 132
Defining Validity 133
Defining Reliability 133
Evaluating a Test 133
Measures of Central Tendency and Variability 135
Derived Scores 137
Identifying Placement on the Normal Curve of Derived Scores 136
Informal Assessment Procedures 136
Familiarizing Yourself with Some Common Tests 137
Assessment of the Individual: More than Just Testing 138
Ethical, Legal, and Professional Vignettes 139

Chapter 13: Multicultural Counseling 142
Diversity in the World 142
The Alligator River: Understanding Our Values 143
Counseling Myths Questionnaire 145
Being "Other" 146
Examining Our Heritage 146
Acknowledging Our Cultural/Ethnic/Religious Affiliation 147
Interviewing a Person from another Cultural Group 147
Experiencing Prejudice 148
Examining the Main Values of Counseling 148
The Culturally Competent Counselor 148

Racist, Sexist, and Culturally Offensive Terms and Jokes 149
Cross-Cultural Counselor Development 149
Multicultural Competence, Advocacy, and Social Justice 151
Identifying Counseling Needs of Clients from Nondominant Groups 152
Counseling Gays and Lesbians 152
Gaining Knowledge about Some Select Groups 153
Ethical, Legal, and Professional Vignettes 154

Chapter 14: Specialty Areas in Counseling 156
Roles and Functions of Counselors 156
Implementation of Roles and Functions 157
Implementing Roles and Functions Using a Developmental Perspective 161
Contrasting the Focus of Counselors in Different Specialty Areas 164
The Use of Counseling Theories in Different Settings 164
Ethical, Legal, and Professional Vignettes 165

Chapter 15: Going To Graduate School, Getting A Job 167
How Did You Get Here? 167
Choosing a Graduate School 167
Applying to Graduate School 167
Finding a Graduate School 168
Finding a Job 169
Role-play Interviewing 170
Creating a Resume 170
Creating a Portfolio 171
Ethical, Legal, and Professional Vignettes 171

REFERENCES 173

APPENDICES
A Perceptions of Ethical Conduct 179
B Cross-Cultural Competencies and Objectives 182
C Advocacy Competencies 186
D Descriptions of Theoretical Orientations and Conceptual Orientation 189
E Clinical Case Report 193
F Consultation at a Mental Health Center 195
G Understanding Your Holland Code 199
H The Normal Curve 203
I Numbers and Percentages of People and Religions in the World 204
J The Graduate Degree Exploration Worksheet 206

INTRODUCTION

Overview

As in the third edition of the workbook, this edition has been designed to offer an experiential learning component to many graduate level courses in a counseling program. The workbook provides exercises in every CACREP required content area, and thus it works well in an introductory survey course. However, because there is a wealth of material available for use in a number of focused content areas, it may also be used in other courses. More specifically, the workbook offers chapters in the following areas:

    Chapter 1:   Counselor Identity
    Chapter 2:   Past, Present, and Future of the Counseling Profession
    Chapter 3:   Standards: Ethics, Accreditation, Credentialing, Multicultural/Advocacy Competencies
    Chapter 4:   Individual Approaches to Counseling
    Chapter 5:   Counseling Skills
    Chapter 6:   Couples and Family Counseling
    Chapter 7:   Group Work
    Chapter 8:   Consultation and Supervision
    Chapter 9:   Human Development: Normal and Abnormal
    Chapter 10: Career Development
    Chapter 11: Research and Evaluation
    Chapter 12: Testing and Assessment
    Chapter 13: Multicultural Counseling
    Chapter 14: Specialty Areas in Counseling
    Chapter 15: Going to Graduate School, Getting a Job

If you are using the workbook along with *The World of the Counselor* text, you will find a natural match between the chapters in the workbook and the sections of the text. More specifically, the chapters in the workbook match the text in the following ways:

Chapters 1, 2, and 3 .... correspond with ... **Section I. Professional Orientation**
Chapters 4 and 5 .... correspond with ... **Section II. Helping Relationship I: Theory and Skills**
Chapters 6, 7, and 8 ... correspond with ... **Section III. Helping Relationship II: The Counselor Working in Systems**
Chapters 9 and 10 .... correspond with ... **Section IV. The Development of the Person**
Chapters 11 and 12 ..... correspond with ... **Section V. Research, Assessment, and Program Evaluation**
Chapter 13 .... corresponds with . **Section VI. Social and Cultural Foundations in Counseling**
Chapter 14 .... corresponds with . **Section VII. Select Specialty Areas**
Chapter 15 .... corresponds with . **Afterword. A Look toward the Future: Applying to Graduate Schools and Finding A Job**

How to Use This Book

Within the workbook you will find a variety of types of experiential learning. A large portion of the workbook relies on small group and class discussion. Many of the exercises are reflective, where you will be asked to think about or write about an event in your life or an important aspect of the counseling relationship. Generally, these exercises can be completed either in class or at home. Some of the exercises require research and/or intensive interviews of individuals and may take a considerable amount of time outside of the classroom.

A few exercises require movement or touch and try to get beyond our usual verbal ways of relating. At the end of each chapter are a number of ethical, legal, and professional vignettes related to the chapter content. When reflecting on these vignettes, you are encouraged to thoroughly read and use as a reference the ethical code of the American Counseling Association, (at www.counseling.org; then click "resources," then "ethics"). You may also want to obtain other ethical guidelines that correspond to the contents of the workbook.

Many of the exercises in the workbook rely on personal disclosure. It is crucial you feel safe if you are to share personal aspects with others. Due to the training of counselor educators, their tendency toward self-disclosure and openness, and the kinds of students that counseling programs tend to attract, it is likely that you will feel comfortable sharing some intimate parts of yourself in class. However, should you feel uncomfortable about self-disclosing in class, please let your instructor know. No student should feel pressured into self-disclosing if he or she does not wish to do so.

Each instructor will have his or her own unique way of using this workbook, and the chapters of the workbook should be used in a manner that corresponds to your instructor's way of teaching. All chapters may not be covered, and instructors will pick and choose exercises that best meet your needs and the needs of the other students in class.

Most of all, have fun with the workbook. You and your instructor should play with the exercises, bend them, change them, extend them, ignore some of them, and integrate your own exercises within the chapters. Please send me copies of your exercises for the next revision of the workbook!

Acknowledgements

First, I'd like to thank Seth Dobrin and Nic Albert from Brooks/Cole publishing for their continued support on all my projects. Also, I am very appreciative of a number of counselors, supervisors and educators whose exercises are dispersed throughout this workbook. Their contributions make this a much stronger workbook. They include: Paula Bickham, Thomas W. Blume, Richmond Calvin, Jane J. Carroll, Jeri Crowell, Montse Casado, Stephanie Dailey, Teresa J. Haase, Cheree Hammond, Amber Lange, Paddy Kennington,; Jered Kolbert, Ken McCurdy, Nicki Nance, Glenda Reynolds, Angela Shores, Gerald Sklare, Darrick Tovar-Murray, Adrian Warren, and Jeffrey Warren.

CHAPTER 1

COUNSELOR IDENTITY: WHAT, WHO, AND HOW

I. Comparing Mental Health Professionals

A. Assessing Differences Among Professionals

We often have varying perceptions of the training, education, and salary of professionals who work in the different social service fields. To evaluate the accuracy of your perceptions for the mental health professional listed in Table 1.1, fill in the items requested and review the answers with your instructor and the rest of the students in class. In completing this exercise, you might want to use *O*NET OnLine* (http://online.onetcenter.org/) or the *Occupational Outlook Handbook* (http://www.bls.gov/oco/), two databases developed by the Department of Labor that provide a large array of information regarding occupational groups.

B. Surveying Differences Through Employment Listings

Obtain a Sunday newspaper and/or a professional magazine that includes want ads (e.g., *Counseling Today*, the *Chronicle of Higher Education*) and examine them for jobs in the social service field. In class, make a list of the job titles, education, training and experience, and salaries being offered. In addition, you may want to compare and contrast jobs for counselors with jobs in other social service fields.

II. Defining Guidance, Counseling, and Psychotherapy

In small groups, or as a class, free associate to the terms *guidance*, *counseling*, and *psychotherapy*. Your instructor will write these associations on the board. Also, place the dictionary definitions of these terms on the board.

1. What differences did you discover among the words *guidance*, *counseling*, and *psychotherapy*?
2. What similarities exist among the words *guidance*, *counseling*, and *psychotherapy*?
3. Discuss with your instructor how your free associations and the dictionary definitions vary from how these terms are used in the profession.

III. Determining Characteristics of the Effective Counselor

The following activities ask you to reflect upon the kinds of qualities, personality characteristics, and skills that you think the effective counselor should embody. Complete this exercise on your own or in small groups.

1. Make a list of the personality characteristics that you believe the effective counselor should embody.
2. Make a list of the skills and techniques that you think the effective counselor should have.
3. What personality characteristics do you think you currently possess that will make you a successful counselor?
4. Choose a person, past or present, historical or fictional, whom you have always admired. What characteristics does (did) this person possess that you believe would be effective within the counseling relationship?

TABLE 1.1 Training, Salary, and Credentialing Differences Among Select Mental Health Professionals

	Education	Type of Courses	Additional Training?	Licensed? (Yes/No)	Salary
Psychologist					
Psychiatrist					
Mental Health Counselor					
School Counselor					
College Counselor					
Rehabilitation Counselor					
Pastoral Counselor					
Social Worker					
Psychotherapist					
Psychiatric Nurse					
Creative Therapist					
Human Service Professional					
Other?					

5. Make a list of those qualities that you believe would be detrimental to the counseling relationship.
6. Figure 1.1 has nine characteristics I believe are important for effective counseling (see Neukrug, 2012). Define each of them as best you can. How similar are they to your list?
7. From all of the qualities you have identified, come up with a final list that you think are critical qualities for effective counseling.

Figure 1.1: Nine Characteristics of the Effective Counselor

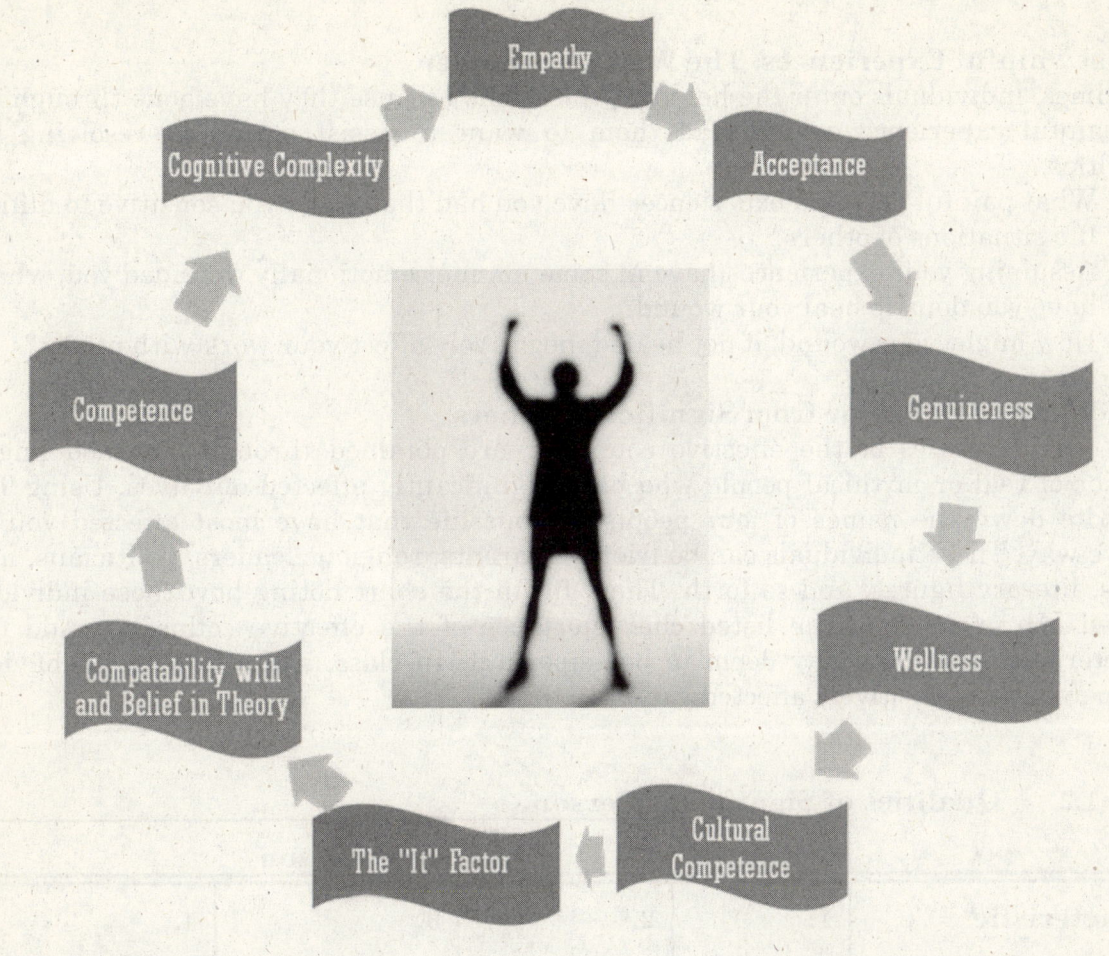

IV. Acquiring the Characteristics of the Effective Counselor

The following sets of questions have to do with how one acquires the qualities of the effective counselor. At home or in class, write down your responses to each item. In class, you will be given the opportunity to discuss your responses in small groups.

A. Influences from the Past
How have the influences listed below affected your desire to enter the counseling field?
1. Parents' education:
2. Parents' occupations:
3. Placement in the family (e.g., middle child, youngest child, etc.):
4. Educational experiences:
5. Work and volunteer experiences:
6. Your values and beliefs:
7. Your religion:
8. Your gender:
9. Your sexual orientation:
10. Your ethnic or cultural background:

11. Developmental milestones (e.g., puberty, first significant relationship, parenting, etc.):
12. Idiosyncratic (unique) experiences:

B. Past Painful Experiences: The Wounded Healer

Oftentimes, individuals enter the helping professions because they have gone through their own painful experience, which lead them to want to assist others in resolving their difficulties.

1. What painful personal experiences have you had that made you sensitive to difficult life situations of others?
2. Assuming your experiences have in some manner emotionally wounded you, what have you done to heal your wound?
3. How might your wound, if not healed, negatively affect your work with others?

C. Modeling of Behavior from Significant Others

Many characteristics of the effective counselor are obtained through our modeling the behavior of real or mythical people who have significantly affected our lives. Using Table 1.2, write down the names of four people in your life that have most affected you in a positive way. These individuals can be friends, parents, religious leaders, politicians, movie figures, literary figures, and so forth. Then, fill in the chart noting how these individuals modeled one or more of the listed characteristics of the effective counselor. Add other characteristics that you may deem to be important. In class, share how the behavior of other persons has positively affected you.

Table 1.2   Qualities of Significant Person

Characteristic ⇓	Significant Person			
	1.	2.	3.	4.
Being Empathic				
Being Accepting				
Being Genuine				
Having a Wellness Focus				
Being Culturally Competent				

Having a Philosophy of Life That Drives How the Person Acts				
Being Competent				
Being Cognitively Complex				
Having "It"— Unique Qualities That Would Make This Person a Good Counselor				
Other Qualities?				

D. Integrating Exercises A, B, & C.
Once you have completed the exercises above, use images, pictures, photos, drawings, or symbols to create a collage depicting your thoughts and reflections of the effective counselor. Share your collages with your peers and be mindful of offering observations about what you see and what you notice, instead of interpretation.

* This exercise was adapted from material by Dr. Teresa J. Haase, Eastern Mennonite University. Her contribution is greatly appreciated.

V. Assessing Self-Development
Directions. The following inventory is designed to assess some of the qualities we just discussed as important to building an effective counseling relationship and tend to increase as a function of age, education, and experience. It is important to answer honestly and to *not fake good* on the instrument. After taking the instrument, your instructor may want to review some of the items on the instrument. The instrument should only be used to give you a rough sense of where you fall in these areas.

Use the scale below when responding to each item.
1. Strongly Agree
2. Slightly Agree
3. Neither Agree nor Disagree
4. Slightly Disagree
5. Strongly Disagree

___1. I believe that my opinions are almost always the correct opinions.
___2. It is usual for people to seek me out to talk about their problems.
___3. I find feedback from a professor enlightening.
___4. The professor almost always has "the answer."

___5. When making decisions, I usually gather information rather than making quick decisions from my "gut."
___6. Usually, when I try to listen to someone, I interject my point of view.
___7. The best type of learning takes place when the professor gives us the facts.
___8. My church, synagogue, or mosque always espouses the right views.
___9. When listening, I usually know from the opening statement what that person is going to say.
___10. I rarely research answers to tough questions.
___11. I can almost always determine the value of a person's belief system based on his or her appearance.
___12. When considering important decisions, it is best to defer to specific figures (e.g., parents) rather than gathering information from multiple sources.
___13. In coming to my views on life, I have spent a lot of time gathering information from others, reflecting, and being introspective.
___14. In understanding other persons with whom I am not familiar, I believe it is important to take the time to listen to them and understand their background.
___15. My views are solid and no one can change them!
___16. I have strong views and usually know what is best for another person when that person is struggling with a difficult situation in life.
___17. I have chosen my values following deep reflection, but I am still open to examining them further.
___18. Through conversations with others, I can change and see the world differently.
___19. When listening to someone, I usually disregard the person's feelings and listen more to "the facts" of the situation.
___20. Generally, I think students can offer much to the knowledge base of a class.
___21. I have rarely questioned the views of my parents.
___22. When in a work group, in an effort to complete tasks efficiently, it is often necessary to make decisions with little or no collaboration.
___23. Most clients need to be given strong advice and firm direction from the beginning of the counseling relationship.
___24. The most important quality of the counseling relationship is understanding how the client comes to make sense of the world.

Scoring the inventory. For items 2, 3, 5, 13, 14, 17, 18, 20, and 24, give yourself $\underline{1}$ point if your response was a "5," $\underline{2}$ points if your response was a "4," $\underline{3}$ points if your response was a "3," $\underline{4}$ points if your response was a "2," and $\underline{5}$ points if your response was a "1." For all other items, give yourself the number of points that you rated the item. The highest score on this inventory is a 120. Higher scores are likely an indication that you are more empathic, accepting, competent, cognitively complex, and open to feedback. Graduate students in counseling usually average around a 95 on this instrument. In class, your instructor might want you to anonymously hand in your score so you can compare it to the rest of the class. This will give you a sense of your score as it compares to your peers.

VI. Am I Ready to Be a Counselor? A Self-Evaluation

Find some time to reflect and respond to the questions below. Then, in class, share in small groups as much as you like and discuss your potential to becoming a counselor.
1. Have I reflected on my professional goals?
2. Have I considered what my reasons are for becoming a counselor?

3. What are my three best qualities and the three areas in my life I need to improve?
4. How would I respond if someone asked me, "What is your philosophy of life?"
5. What is my belief about the underlying nature of people (e.g., people are born good, bad, neutral, etc.)?
6. How well do I manage work-related stress?
7. How do I balance work and personal time?
8. How effectively do I handle feedback from others?
9. What role do my gender, religion, sexual orientation, and ethnic values play in my life?
10. Am I able to embrace all aspects of a counselor's job in a timely fashion (paperwork, meetings, etc.)?
11. Considering the nine characteristics of effective counselors noted earlier, which one is my strength and which is my weakness?
12. How do my answers to the questions above detract or add to my goal of becoming a counselor?

* This exercise was adapted from material by Dr. Glenda Reynolds, Auburn University at Montgomery. Her contribution is greatly appreciated.

VII. Learning about Professional Associations
A. The American Counseling Association and Its Affiliates
1. Become familiar with the American Counseling Association. Some ways you may do this is to:
   a. Go to the ACA website, www.counseling.org
   b. Look up ACA in the *Encyclopedia of Associations*
   c. Contact ACA by phone at 1-800-347-6647 or by email at membership@cousneling.org, and ask them to send you information
   d. Ask your instructor if he or she has information concerning ACA

2. Gather information about and discuss the purpose and function of each of the divisions of ACA as listed below (links to their websites can be obtained through the "Division Link" at www.counseling.org). Which association(s) would you consider joining? Why?
   - AACE: Association for Assessment in Counseling
   - AADA: Association for Adult Development and Aging
   - ACC: Association for Creativity in Counseling
   - ACCA: American College Counseling Association
   - ACEG: Association for Counselors and Educators in Government
   - ACES: Association for Counselor Education and Supervision
   - ALGBTIC: Association for Lesbian, Gay, Bisexual, and Transgender Issues in Counseling
   - AGLBIC: Association for Gay, Lesbian, and Bisexual Issues in Counseling
   - AMCD: Association for Multicultural Counseling and Development
   - AMHCA: American Mental Health Counselors Association
   - ARCA: American Rehabilitation Counseling Association
   - ASCA: American School Counselor Association
   - ASERVIC: Association for Spiritual, Ethical & Religious Values in Counseling
   - ASGW: Association for Specialists in Group Work
   - C-AHEAD: Counseling Association for Humanistic Education and Development
   - CSJ: Counselors for Social Justice

- IAAOC: International Association of Addiction and Offender Counselors
- IAMFC: International Association of Marriage and Family Counselors
- NCDA: National Career Development Association
- NECA: National Employment Counseling Association

3. Gather information and discuss the purpose and function of each of the following associations and organizations that work with the American Counseling Association (information about these affiliates can be obtained from clicking on the "About Us" link and then the "Professional Partners" link at www.counseling.org):
   - The ACA Insurance Trust (ACAIT)
   - The American Counseling Association Foundation (ACAF)
   - The Council on Accreditation of Counseling and Related Programs (CACREP)
   - The National Board for Certified Counselors (NBCC)
   - Chi Sigma Iota

4. Join a Counseling Interest Network or Listserv
   - Join one of ACA's many interest networks by clicking "Interest Networks" at www.counseling.org
   - Join the graduate student listserv (COUNSGRADS) or the Diversegrad-L, which discusses diversity issues in counseling by clicking on "Listservs" at www.counseling.org
   - If you're a doctoral student or interested in issues in counselor education and supervision, join CESNET-L at https://listserv.kent.edu/cgi-bin/wa.exe?SUBED1=CESNET-L&A=1

B. Other Professional Associations

The following lists a number of professional associations in the social services along with their websites. Visit some or all of their websites and share information in class about them:

- AAMFT (Am. Association of Marriage and Family Therapy) (www.aamft.org)
- AAPC (American Association of Pastoral Counselors) (www.aapc.org)
- AATA (American Art Therapy Association) (www.arttherapy.org)
- ACPA (College Students Educators International) (www.myacpa.org)
- ADTA (American Dance Therapy Association) (www.adta.org)
- AMTA (American Music Therapy Association) (www.musictherapy.org)
- APA (American Psychiatric Association) (www.psych.org)
- APA (American Psychological Association) (www.apa.org)
- APNA (American Psychiatric Nurses Association) (www.apna.org)
- APsaA (American Psychoanalytical Association) (www.apsa.org/)
- APT (Association for Play Therapy) (www.a4pt.org/)
- NASP (National Association of School Psychologist) (www.nasponline.org)
- NASW (National Association of Social Workers) (www.socialworkers.org)
- NOHS (National Org. for Human Services) (www.nationalhumanservices.org)
- NRCA (National Rehabilitation Counselors Association) (www.nrca-net.org/)

C. General Information about Professional Associations
1. Discuss in class some of the benefits you uncovered when one joins various professional associations.
2. Today, most professional journals in the field of counseling can be accessed online (your reference librarian should be able to help you access them). By going online or by going to your library, obtain copies of some articles from professional journals and share them in class. Compare and contrast the kinds of articles from the various journals.
3. Obtain membership applications from your professor or online at the associations' website. Share membership applications. Join.
4. Ask your professor and/or professionals in the field to share knowledge of local conferences and/or workshops sponsored by professional associations. Attend the workshop or conference and share the information with your class.
5. Ask your professor and/or professionals in the field to share knowledge of any local branches or affiliates of state or national professional associations (e.g., there may be a local branch of your state counseling association). Join the association, attend workshops, and become active on their board. Share this information in class.

VIII. Advocating for Our Profession

When we advocate for our profession, we are also shaping our professional identity. Advocating includes such things as making phone calls to officials, writing letters or sending e-mails to politicians and others, recruiting additional counselors in the cause, donating money to causes, joining professional associations who hire professional lobbyists with your dues, and so forth. For this exercise, identify a cause in the profession, and in small groups, present this issue to the class. Discuss why this issue is significant and the consequence of counselors not achieving this goal. Discuss the ramifications of counselors being poor professional advocates. What do you believe will increase counselors' motivation to be better advocates? What can you personally do to become a profession advocate? To help you pick a cause, you may want to go to http://capwiz.com/counseling/home/.

* This exercise was adapted from material by Dr. Amber Lange, the University of Toledo. Her contribution is greatly appreciated.

IX. Interviewing Professionals in the Field

Using the list of questions below as a guideline, have different students in the class interview a wide range of mental health professionals (e.g., human service professional, family therapist, social worker, psychologist, psychiatrist, psychiatric nurse, school counselor, clinical mental health counselor, college counselor, rehabilitation counselor, etc.). In small groups, discuss the similarities and differences you find among the professionals. During your interview, discuss the following questions:
1. Why the professional decided to enter the chosen profession
2. What degree(s) was (were) obtained
3. The "theoretical" orientation of the professional
4. The job roles and functions as defined by the professional
5. His or her entry-level salary
6. His or her current salary
7. His or her view on the differences between the varying helping professions
8. The professional association(s) to which he or she belongs

X. Conducting a Detailed Analysis of an Agency Where Counselors Work

Using the guidelines that follow, interview a counselor in a specialty area of your choice (e.g., elementary school counseling, community agency/mental health counseling, college counseling, and so forth). Discuss what you found in class.

Guidelines (Describe the Following)

1. The name and address of setting (e.g., mental health center, high school, college counseling center)
2. The number of total staff at the setting
3. The number and type of administrative staff (e.g., principal, assistant principal, clinical director, medical director, director, etc.)
4. The approximate salaries of administrative staff
5. The number of "direct service" personnel (mental health professionals who work with clients)
6. The types of direct service personnel (e.g., school counselors, outpatient therapists, mental health aids, supervisors, program coordinators, group leaders, family counselors, etc.)
7. The degrees held by direct service personnel
8. The ethnic/cultural diversity of direct service personnel
9. The approximate salaries of direct service personnel
10. The number and type of support staff (e.g., secretaries, clerical staff, etc.)
11. Whether the setting is private or public
12. The funding of the setting
13. The policy and practices statement (a written statement that explains the functions of the setting and the roles of the staff)
14. The type of clients seen (e.g., high school students, adults dealing with adjustment issues, individuals with mental illness, etc.)
15. The diversity of clients seen
16. How the clients are obtained
17. The process whereby the client initially contacts the counseling office
18. The process that describes how clients are diagnosed, needs are assessed, goals are established, referrals are made, and follow-up is accomplished
19. The payment process
20. The types of counseling and assistance that takes place (e.g., individual, group, family, etc.)
21. The typical length of counseling/interviewing sessions
22. The typical kind of paperwork necessary for counselors to complete
23. The typical number of hours, days, weeks, months, or years that a client would spend with a counselor at the setting
24. The manner in which clients are typically terminated
25. The manner in which the setting evaluates itself
26. The staff development effort (in-house workshops, guest speakers, monetary support for conferences, etc.)
27. How the setting deals with ethical concerns related to confidentiality, competence, and training in multicultural counseling
28. Whether the policy and practices statement matches what is actually going on at the setting

29. Whether any recent or foreseen future trends have affected or may affect the ways in which the counselor does his or her work at this setting
30. Other comments

XI. Ethical, Legal, and Professional Vignettes

(The ACA's code is at www.counseling.org under "Resources"). In responding to the following, consider referring to the ACA's code.

At the end of each workbook chapter, you will find a series of ethical and professional vignettes specifically focused on the chapter content. Please read them and respond to the questions that follow. If appropriate, review the ACA ethical code when making your response, and identify what section of the code addresses the vignette. Also, feel free to refer to other ethical codes. In many cases, the response will not be clear-cut, and there may not be a "correct" answer. In addition, the responses may vary depending on specific laws within your state. Remember, these vignettes are intended to stimulate thought and generate discussion.

1. As counselors we have a professional responsibility to confront our colleagues if we believe they are acting unethically. Sometimes, this is more difficult than it seems. For instance, ponder the following:
   a. Think about an important concern you may not have shared with a friend and approach him or her.
   b. Consider confronting a professor on his or her teaching style or assignments if you believe there is reason for improvement.
   c. Consider talking to a family member about some unfinished business you might have with him or her.
2. At a local workshop, a colleague of yours responds to a question in the audience regarding the training of social workers. Your colleague states, "Well, they can be perfectly nice people, but their training is certainly far from adequate." Is this ethical? Is this legal? Is this professional? Should you say anything?
3. In making a decision on a particularly difficult ethical dilemma, a colleague of yours decides to use the APA code of ethics as it seems to concur more closely with the decision he is making. In fact, the ACA code would advise the colleague not to make the decision. Is your colleague acting ethically? Professionally? Legally? Should you do anything?
4. You discover that a counselor is working outside of his area of competence. You report him to the ethics committees of ACA and to your state counseling association. It turns out that he is not a member of either association. Have you acted ethically and professionally? Are there any legal actions you can take? Do you have any other alternatives? Should you speak directly to the counselor?
5. A colleague of yours, who has a master's degree in counseling and works at a local agency, often refers to himself as a "psychologist" when talking with friends. Is this ethical? Is this legal?
6. As a school counselor, your guidance director tells you that you must work in a directive fashion with your students. None of this "empathy stuff" or "Rogerian nonsense," she says. It is your job, she states, to be active and directive with your clients if they are going to succeed in school. Is she acting ethically? Legally? What should you do?

7. A friend of yours is a social worker and tells you she is doing career counseling with her clients. You are aware that she has no training in career counseling. What should you do?
8. You've just finished graduate school, and one of your classmates says, "Now that I'm finished, I can finally do what I want to do: in-depth analytical work with my clients." Is this ethical? Legal? Professional? What, if anything, should you say to this person?
9. You believe that a colleague of yours is doing ineffective counseling because he has not worked through some of his own issues. What should you do?
10. A colleague advertises herself as a psychotherapist. Is this ethical? Legal? Professional?
11. Following the attainment of her degree, a counselor takes advanced training in a new in-depth therapeutic approach. She then opens a practice in which she applies this training. She is not licensed. Can she practice without a license? Can she practice this kind of training?
12. You discover that a social services employee who has his degree in human services is calling himself a counselor. Is this ethical? Professional? Legal? Should you do anything? Can you do anything?

CHAPTER 2

THE COUNSELING PROFESSION'S PAST, PRESENT, AND FUTURE

I: Important Names and Places

Organized loosely by year, the following is a list of select persons, events, concepts, and organizations that greatly affected the development of the counseling profession. From your text and any additional research that you might conduct, write a brief statement that describes the historical importance of each item listed. At the end of this list, add any other items that you believe are relevant to the development of the counseling profession.

1. 3000 BCE Ancient Egypt _____
2. Hippocrates _____
3. Plato _____
4. Aristotle _____
5. Poltonius _____
6. Augustine _____
7. Thomas Aquinas _____
8. Sanchez de Arevalo _____
9. Elizabethan Poor Laws _____
10. Descartes _____
11. John Locke _____
12. James Mill _____
13. Phillipe Pinel _____
14. Benjamin Rush _____
15. Anton Mesmer _____
16. Charity Organization Societies _____
17. Jean Martin Charcot _____
18. Dorothea Dix _____
19. Wilhelm Wundt _____
20. Sir Francis Galton _____
21. Sigmund Freud _____
22. G. Stanley Hall _____
23. James Cattell _____

24. John Dewey_____
25. Alfred Binet_____
26. Jane Addams_____
27. Emil Kraepelin_____
28. Pierre Janet_____
29. Ivan Pavlov_____
30. William James_____
31. Mary Richmond_____
32. Eli Weaver_____
33. Jesse Davis_____
34. Anna Reed_____
35. Frank Parsons_____
36. Clifford Beers_____
37. NVGA_____
38. Army Alpha Test_____
39. Woodworth Personal Data Sheet_____
40. Strong Interest Inventory_____
41. E.G. Williamson_____
42. John Brewer_____
43. B.F. Skinner_____
44. Wagner O'Day Act_____
45. American Psychiatric Association_____
46. Carl Rogers_____
47. Division 17 of APA_____
48. New Approaches to Counseling (1960s)_____
49. APGA_____
50. NASW_____
51. NDEA_____
52. 1st Diagnostic and Statistical Manual_____
53. Community Mental Health Centers Act_____
54. Great Society Initiatives_____
55. 1973 Rehabilitation Act_____

56. CORE_____
57. PL94-142 and IDEA_____
58. *Donaldson v. O'Connor*_____
59. Cross-Cultural Issues First Identified_____
60. "Microcounseling Skills Training"_____
61. NACMHC_____
62. CACREP_____
63. NBCC_____
64. AACD_____
65. ACA_____
66. ASCA_____
67. AMHCA_____
68. AMCD_____
69. "Other" ACA Divisions_____
70. Expansion of Credentialing_____
71. Multicultural Counseling Competencies_____
72. Advocacy Competencies_____
73. ASCA National Model_____
74. Current ACA Ethics Code_____
75. Newest CACREP Standards_____
76. Evidence-Based Practice_____
77. Crisis, Disaster, and Trauma Training_____
78. 20/20: A Vision for the Future_____
79. Other_____
80. Other_____

II: Are There Shamans Amongst Us?

Many religious and cultural traditions have a rich history that includes the use of wise men and women, sometimes called shamans. In class, have students share what personal knowledge they may have regarding the place that shamans have played within religious and/or cultural traditions. Then discuss how the values and concepts expressed by the shamans you identified are similar or different from core values inherent in the counseling profession.

III: What We Can Learn from Great People of History
A. Identifying Positive Qualities
Using the list of great people in history that follows, describe those personal characteristics that each person may have embodied that could be considered vital elements to the counseling relationship. Feel free to add other names to the list:

Jesus	Moses	Muhammad
Gandhi	Martin Luther King, Jr.	Eleanor Roosevelt
Joan of Arc	Abraham Lincoln	Dorothy Day
Mother Theresa	Malcolm X	Bishop Tutu
Nelson Mandela	Amelia Earhart	Others?

B. Role-Playing
Your instructor will ask you to break into small groups and identify one individual to be the "counselor." The rest of the group should play a dysfunctional family, work group, or counseling group. Have the counselor intervene with the group by modeling the qualities listed from Exercise A.

C. Identifying One's Weaker Qualities
Make a list of qualities with which each individual in Exercise A may have struggled (skeletons in the closet!). If no one in class can identify some qualities for each person listed, you might consider researching the individual in more detail. Consider how each of these people was considered great, yet struggled with his or her issues. Discuss how a counselor can model effective counseling skills, embrace qualities considered positive for the counseling relationship, and still make mistakes at times—not be perfect within the counseling relationship.

IV: Learning from Related Mental Health Professions
Compare and contrast the histories of the varying mental health professions (e.g., counseling, social work, psychology) and discuss how each impacted the counseling profession.

V. Historical Influences on Job Choice
A: Interviewing Professionals in Related Mental Health Disciplines
Using the list of questions below as a guideline, have one-fourth of the class interview a human service professional, one-fourth a social worker, one-fourth a psychologist, and the remainder a counselor (of course, feel free to interview other professionals also):
1. Why did he or she decide to enter the chosen profession?
2. Why did the individual choose his or her profession as opposed to one of the others?
3. What degree(s) did he or she obtain?
4. Is there anything about the core values of this individual's profession that led him or her to choose this degree over other ones?
5. What is the theoretical orientation of the professional?
6. What are the job roles and functions as defined by the professional?
7. What was his or her entry-level salary?
8. What is his or her current salary?
9. What is his or her view on the differences and similarities among the different professions?

10. What functions and roles of this professional are inherent in the history of the discipline (e.g., the fact that many counselors have expertise and conduct career counseling because the origins of the profession are in vocational counseling)?

B. Comparing Professions

After having interviewed individuals from the four professions in Exercise A, the class should break into groups of four students, with each group having one student representing each of the disciplines. Then discuss the following questions:
1. What similarities and differences did you find among the professions?
2. Did you find differences among the professions as a function of their diverse histories?
3. What positive and negative aspects could you deduct from each of the professions?

VI. A Look toward the Future

A. The Use of Computers
1. **Social Networking and Listservs**
    a. How do you believe social networking (e.g., Facebook) has, and will continue to affect, the counseling profession?
    b. Do you believe it's ethical to seek out a client's social network presence (e.g. Facebook page) without him or her knowing about it?
    c. Discuss and consider joining the following Listservs:
        i. *COUNSGRADS* (for graduate students in counseling) (go to http://www.counseling.org/ and click "Students")
        ii. *Diversegrad-L* (for counselors interested in diversity issues) (go to http://www.counseling.org/ and click "Students")
        iii. *CESNET-L* (for issues related to counselor education, supervision, advanced study, and research) (go to https://listserv.kent.edu/cgi-bin/wa.exe?SUBED1=CESNET-L&A=1)

2. **The Use of Computers with Clients and in Research and Assessment**
    a. In small groups, discuss the trend for personal computers to be used for testing, billing, diagnosis, and case report writing. What privacy issues are involved in such use?
    b. Increasingly, students no longer need to go to the library to find articles and other research materials as a vast majority can be accessed through the Internet. Discuss how this changes the nature of doing research.
    c. Assessment of clients can now be completed on the Internet or on personal computers. Discuss privacy issues related to such assessment.

3. **Counseling Online**
    a. In small groups, discuss your thoughts about online counseling.
    b. Review the ACA ethical code, section A.12, for the use of electronic communications over the Internet and examine how it deals with counseling online. Discuss in small groups and in class.

4. **Distance Learning and Online Counseling Programs**
   a. CACREP has accredited some counseling programs that are predominantly online or are taught through distance learning. What are the advantages and disadvantages to this trend?
   b. What courses, if any, do you believe are more amenable to being offered online or through distance learning?

5. **Webpages**
   a. Examine the webpages below and have an in-class discussion comparing and contrasting them:
      1. ACA: (American Counseling Association) (www.counseling.org/)
      2. ACA's Divisions (Go to www.counseling.org and click "Divisions")
      3. AAMFT: (Am. Assoc. of Marriage and Family Therapy) (www.aamft.org/)
      4. NOHS: (National Org. of Human Service) (www.nationalhumanservices.org/)
      5. NASW: (National Association of Social Workers) (www.naswdc.org/)
      6. APA: (American Psychological Association) (www.apa.org)
      7. APA: (American Psychiatric Association) (www.psych.org/)
      8. APNA: (American Psychiatric Nurses Association) (www.apna.org/)
      9. AATA: (American Art Therapy Association) (www.arttherapy.org/)
      10. AAPC (American Association of Pastoral Counselors (http://aapc.org/)

B. HMOs, PPOs, EAPs, and National Health Care Coverage

In small groups, research and/or discuss the terms Health Maintenance Organizations (HMOs), Preferred Provider Organizations (PPOs), Employee Assistance Programs (EAPs), and/or traditional health insurance plans. Compare and contrast their mental health delivery systems in the following ways:
1. What services tend to be offered by each?
2. Does an individual need to go through a primary care physician to receive services?
3. Is preventive care covered?
4. Are mental health services covered?
5. What limitations are there toward covered mental health services?
6. What mental health providers are covered under the plan (e.g., LPCs, psychologists, LCSWs, etc.)?
7. What is the payment for mental health services? Is there a difference based on degree?
8. What impact does the national health care law have on the delivery of mental health services?

C. Standard of Practice

Standards of practice have increasingly become critical to the effective delivery of counseling services. Discuss how each of the following has and will continue to impact the counseling profession:
1. The use of informed consent protocols and professional disclosure statements
2. Multicultural Counseling Competencies
3. Advocacy Competencies
4. Credentialing
5. Increased use of supervision
6. Ethical codes

D. Advances in Medicine
Discuss how the following medical breakthroughs might affect the counseling profession:
1. New psychotropic medications
2. Advances in genetic research
3. Use of biological interventions to treat mental health problems (e.g., brain surgery, modern-day electric shock treatment for depression, light therapy, brain stimulation)
4. Advances in the use of holistic health approaches

E. Complementary, Alternative, and Integrative
Complementary medicine or therapy includes products, systems, or practices used in conjunction with conventional methods to treat biological and mental health problems. Alternative therapy is when alternative approaches are used instead of conventional methods. An integrative approach suggests that traditional healing methods are integrated with complementary or alternative approaches.
1. Discuss this increasing focus in the counseling profession with particular emphasis on its efficacy—Do you think it works? What evidence is there?
2. Would you be willing to use these approaches?
3. What training would you need, and how would you gain it?

VII: Are We Ready for Another "Paradigm Shift?"
Major advances are often the result of a "paradigm shift" in the manner in which the world is viewed. This shift occurs because knowledge builds on prior knowledge and the time is ripe for a synthesis of this prior knowledge and the development of new, revolutionary ways of understanding what has come before. For instance, the development of psychoanalysis was a paradigm shift in how the world viewed personality development. Other paradigm shifts have included the widespread use of psychotropic medications, the growing belief that mental health problems may be at least partially biologically rooted, and the growing tendency for clinicians to be "integrative" or "eclectic."
1. Do you believe the mental health professions are primed for a paradigm shift?
2. If yes, in what direction do you think it would take? If no, why not?

VIII. Keeping Yourself Well in a High Stress Occupation
One method of assessing your level of wellness is by examining what Myers and Sweeney (2008) identify as the indivisible self. This model views wellness as a primary factor composed of five subfactors that encompass 17 wellness dimensions that are dispersed among the five subfactors. These factors include the creative self, coping self, social self, essential self, and physical self. This model also takes into account the individual's context.

Using Table 2.1 as your guide, complete an informal assessment on each of the factors to determine what areas you might want to address in your life. For instance, score yourself from 1 to 5 on each of the subfactors, with 5 indicating the area you most need to work on. Then, find the average for each of the five factors. Next, write down the ways you can better yourself in any factor where your scores seem problematic (probably scores of 3, 4, or 5). You may also want to consider how the contextual elements affect your ability for you to embrace a wellness perspective. For a more extensive review of your wellness, see Myers and Sweeney (2008).

Table 2.1: Abbreviated Definitions of Components of the Indivisible Self Model

Wellness Factor	Definition
Total Wellness	The sum of all items on the 5F-Wel; a measure of one's general well-being or total wellness
Creative Self	The combination of attributes that each of us forms to make a unique place among others in our social interactions and to positively interpret our world
Thinking	Being mentally active, open-minded; having the ability to be creative and experimental; having a sense of curiosity, a need to know and to learn; the ability to solve problems
Emotions	Being aware of or in touch with one's feelings; being able to experience and express one's feelings appropriately, both positive and negative
Control	Belief that one can usually achieve the goals one sets for oneself; having a sense of a plan in life; being able to be assertive in expressing one's needs
Work	Being satisfied with one's work; having adequate financial security; feeling that one's skills are used appropriately; the ability to cope with workplace stress
Positive Humor	Being able to laugh at one's own mistakes and the unexpected things that happen; the ability to use humor to accomplish even serious tasks
Coping Self	The combination of elements that regulate one's responses to life events and provide a means to transcend the negative effects of these events
Leisure	Activities done in one's free time; satisfaction with one's leisure activities; having at least one activity in which "I lose myself and time stands still"
Stress Management	General perception of one's own self-management or self-regulation; seeing change as an opportunity for growth; ongoing self-monitoring and assessment of one's coping resource
Self-Worth	Accepting who and what one is, positive qualities along with imperfections; valuing oneself as a unique individual
Realistic Beliefs	Understanding that perfection and being loved by everyone are impossible goals, and having the courage to be imperfect
Social Self	Social support through connections with others in friendships and intimate relationships, including family ties
Friendship	Social relationships that involve a connection with others individually or in community, but that do not have a marital, sexual, or familial commitment; having friends in whom one can trust and who can provide emotional, material, or informational support when needed
Love	The ability to be intimate, trusting, and self-disclosing with another person; having a family or family-like support system characterized by shared spiritual values, the ability to solve conflict in a mutually respectful way, healthy communication styles, and mutual appreciation
Essential Self	Essential meaning-making processes in relation to life, self, and others
Spirituality	Personal beliefs and behaviors that are practiced as part of the recognition that a person is more than the material aspects of mind and body
Gender Identity	Satisfaction with one's gender; feeling supported in one's gender; transcendence of gender identity (i.e., ability to be androgynous)
Cultural Identity	Satisfaction with one's cultural identity; feeling supported in one's cultural identity; transcendence of one's cultural identity
Self-Care	Taking responsibility for one's wellness through self-care and safety habits that are preventive in nature; minimizing the harmful effects of pollution in one's environment
Physical Self	The biological and physiological processes that compose the physical aspects of a person's development and functioning
Exercise	Engaging in sufficient physical activity to keep in good physical condition; maintaining flexibility through stretching
Nutrition	Eating a nutritionally balanced diet, maintaining a normal weight (i.e., within 15% of the ideal), and avoiding overeating
Contexts	
Local context	Systems in which one lives most often—families, neighborhoods, and communities—and one's perceptions of safety in these systems
Institutional context	Social and political systems that affect one's daily functioning and serve to empower or limit development in obvious and subtle ways, including education, religion, government, and the media
Global context	Factors such as politics, culture, global events, and the environment that connect one to others around the world
Chronometrical context	Growth, movement, and change in the time dimension that are perpetual, of necessity positive, and purposeful

Source: Myers, J., & Sweeney, T. J. (2008). Wellness counseling: The evidence base and practice. *Journal of Counseling and Development, 86*, p. 485.

IX. Ethical, Legal, and Professional Vignettes (The ACA's code is at www.counseling.org under "Resources"). In responding to the following, consider referring to the ACA's code.

1. A colleague of yours tells you that he is practicing "animal magnetism," a practice from the late 1800s in which individuals lie in tubs and iron filings were placed over them. A trained expert would then assist the individual in ridding him or her of psychological problems. What should you say to your friend? What should you do?
2. A counselor tells you that she is practicing phrenology, the age-old practice of determining psychological and cognitive functioning from the shape of one's head. You ask her if there is evidence that this practice works, and she says, "It's been around for centuries, obviously it holds some truth." What should you say to your friend? What should you do?
3. A classmate of yours tells you that she is involved in "New Age" therapy, particularly the use of flower extracts in the healing process. She sells these extracts to her clients and uses them as an adjunct to counseling. Is this ethical? Is this legal? Is this reasonable? What should you do?
4. You have heard that there is a new therapeutic technique that may be effective in working with clients who have obsessive-compulsive disorder. You are interested in using it. What precautions should you take before practicing it?
5. With the advent of Health Maintenance Organizations (HMOs) and the push in schools for briefer modes of counseling, you realize that you must change the approach to counseling you have been practicing. You have been using an approach that has historically been shown to work with a wide range of clients, and you are not convinced that the brief counseling approach you have been asked to use will show the same efficacy with all types of clients. How should you proceed?
6. A psychiatrist you know continues to use psychodynamic therapy with some clients for whom the approach has been shown to not be very effective. Is this ethical? Professional? Legal? What should you do?
7. You discover that a colleague of yours is offering counseling services through a website. From the website, individuals can go into chat rooms and discuss their problems with a licensed counselor. "Clients" are charged for their services online. Is this ethical? Professional? Legal? What should you do?
8. A friend of yours is a staunch advocate for holistic health methods and states that living a healthy lifestyle can help all mental health problems. She does not believe in the use of medication and will not refer to a psychiatrist under any circumstances. Is this ethical? Professional? Legal? What should you do?
9. You know a counselor who is beginning to refer clients with severe depression for electroshock treatment. Is this ethical and legal? What precautions, if any, should be taken?
10. You discover that a fellow student found a website that will conduct a literature review on a counseling-related subject for a fee. He has decided to use this site for a literature review for a paper he is writing. Is this ethical? Professional? Legal? What should you do?

11. You discover that a counselor who works for an Employee Assistance Program (EAP) has a bias against referring employees for counseling, even if they may need it. The EAP counselor is concerned that if he makes too many referrals, he may lose his job because referrals are costly to the company. Is this ethical? Professional? Legal? What, if anything, should the counselor do?
12. A counselor with whom you work has obtained her degree from an online, non-CACREP-accredited counseling program. Should you express concerns about her abilities? Would your concerns be any different than concerns about any student who did not graduate from a CACREP-accredited program? Are CACREP-accredited programs inherently better?
13. You are concerned about a colleague of yours because she constantly seems under stress. You wonder if her stress level results in inadequate client care. You decide to talk with her, and she tells you that she works out four or five days a week and she believes the exercise relieves her stress. You are doubtful and believe she is still very highly stressed. What, if anything, should you do?
14. A counselor to whom you periodically refer tells you he refuses to work with clients who are diagnosed as having a "personality disorder." He states that they are too difficult to work with, and he believes that such clients would simply drain him of energy and take away from his ability to work with other clients. In addition, he tells you that few insurance companies will reimburse for individuals with this diagnosis. He does, however, find appropriate referrals for these clients. Has he acted ethically? Professionally? Morally?

CHAPTER 3

STANDARDS IN THE PROFESSION: ETHICS, ACCREDITATION, CREDENTIALING, AND MULTICULUTRAL AND ADVOCACY COMPETENCIES

PART I: ETHICS

I. Developing Ethical Guidelines

In small groups, consider the kinds of items you would include if you were developing an ethical code for counselors. In your discussion, take the following into account:
1. Values that may be unique to counselors and the counseling profession
2. Societal values that you believe should be included in the guidelines
3. Universal moral values that you believe should be included in the guidelines
4. How you might address major differences in values and morality among individuals (e.g., those who might be pro-choice versus those who might be pro-life)
5. Differences in values of various ethnic and cultural groups in the United States (Latinas/Latinos African Americans, Whites, Males, Females, etc.)

II. Challenging Ethical Beliefs

As defined by the ACA ethical code, the list below contains issues that are considered to be an ethical violation some or all of the time. For each issue, (1) identify where in the ethical guideline the issue is addressed and how it may be an ethical violation (see the ACA's code by clicking "Resources" at www.counseling.org), (2) present an understanding of why you believe the profession has chosen to view this issue as unethical some or all of the time, and (3) develop a scenario where you could argue that acting in such a manner could potentially be beneficial to a client.

Issues
1. Counseling a friend or neighbor
2. Not informing your client of the rules of the counseling relationship
3. Allowing a client to be verbally attacked within a group setting
4. Having sex with a client
5. Having a romantic relationship with a friend or relative of a client
6. Breaking confidentiality when the guidelines indicate one should not
7. Allowing a client to commit suicide
8. Revealing client information gained through testing to a third party
9. Concealing information from the parents of a child whom you are seeing in counseling, despite the fact that they requested such information
10. Attending the wedding of a client

III. Perceptions of Ethical Behaviors

Appendix A provides a survey you can take to examine 77 counselor behaviors. Take the survey to assess which of those behaviors you believe are ethical and also to examine how strongly you feel about your decision. Then, in class, discuss your results with other students. If you would like to compare your results to a random sample of ACA members, see Neukrug, E., & Milliken, T. (2011). Counselors' perceptions of ethical behaviors. *Journal of Counseling and Development 89*, 206-216.

IV. Violating Ethics: The Consequences

Contact each of the associations or boards listed below and determine whether or not they are empowered to deal with ethical complaints. If they are, find out exactly what they can do if they find that an ethical violation has taken place.
1. Your state licensing board for counselors
2. Your state counseling association
3. The American Counseling Association
4. The National Board for Certifying Counselors (NBCC)
5. Related professional associations and licensing boards (e.g., APA, State licensing board of social workers)

V. Malpractice Insurance

Contact your professional association (e.g., ACA, ASCA, AMHCA, ACCA) and examine the kind of malpractice insurance it offers. Report what you find in class. Pay particular attention to the following:
1. Is insurance offered for private practice?
2. Is insurance offered for working in a privately run agency?
3. Is insurance offered for working in a public-funded agency?
4. Is insurance offered if you work part time?
5. Is insurance offered for graduate students?
6. Are there separate rates as a function of the type of counseling one conducts (school counselor, college counselor, mental health counselor)?

PART II: ACCREDITATION

VI. Developing Accreditation Standards

In small groups or as a class, consider what you would require of a counseling program if you were an accreditation body charged with developing accreditation standards.

Specifically, speak to each of the following:
1. Admissions requirements
2. Curriculum
3. Number of credits
4. Faculty/student ratio
5. Minimum number of full-time faculty
6. Minimum full-time to adjunct faculty ratio
7. Number of total hours for internship (of these, how many would be direct service?)
8. Comprehensive exam and/or thesis
9. Acceptability of online or distance learning courses
10. How you might assess the program
11. Other?

VII. Reviewing CACREP's Accreditation Standards

Have your instructor make available the CACREP accreditation standards, or go to www.cacrep.org and find the link for the most recent standards. Your instructor can assign various aspects of the standards to small groups. After reviewing the standards in your small groups, do the following:
1. Summarize and present various aspects of the standards in class.
2. Using the standards as a reference, critically evaluate your counseling program.
3. Make suggestions for change in your counseling program as a result of your critical review in "b."
4. Critically review the standards. What makes sense? What could be changed?

VIII. Accreditation of Related Professional Associations

Your instructor will have the class separate into smaller groups, and each group will be assigned a professional organization to research its accreditation process. Each group can present a short summary of this process to class. Below are some possible professional groups:

1. Psychiatrists
2. Counseling Psychologists
3. Clinical Psychologists
4. School Psychologists
5. Social Workers
6. Human Service Professionals
7. Pastoral Counselors
8. Psychiatric Nurses
9. Art Therapists
10. Rehabilitation counselors

PART III: CREDENTIALING

IX. Registration, Certification, and Licensing: What Are the Differences?

Discuss the differences between registration, certification, and licensing by doing the following:
1. Ask in class if anyone is registered, certified, or licensed in any field. What did he or she have to do to gain this credential?
2. Interview credentialed professionals, and ask them what they did to become credentialed. Compare and contrast professionals and credentialing processes.
3. Contact the Board of Education and the counselor licensing board in your state. Find out what a person has to do to become a credentialed school counselor or licensed professional counselor.

X. Comparing Credentialing Processes

Table 3.1 lists a number of mental health professionals. Using the six questions that follow, place the answer to each question in the spaces provided across from the corresponding number in the table. For example, in the first row, where it says "school counselor," across from number "1," I would want to state whether or not school counselors have a credentialing process and what kind it is. For item "2," I would state who regulates the credentialing process, if one exists. And so forth. In some cases, more than one credentialing process exists, so be as thorough as possible.

Table 3.1: Credentialing Comparisons of Mental Health Professionals

School Counselor	1. 2. 3. 4. 5.
Agency/Mental Health Counselor	1. 2. 3. 4. 5.
College Counselor	1. 2. 3. 4. 5.
Creative Therapist (Eg., Art Therapist)	1. 2. 3. 4. 5.
Psychotherapist	1. 2. 3. 4. 5.
Psychiatric Nurse	1. 2. 3. 4. 5.
Human Service Professional	1. 2. 3. 4. 5.
Social Worker	1. 2. 3. 4. 5.
Psychologist	1. 2. 3. 4. 5.
Psychiatrist	1. 2. 3. 4. 5.

1. Does a credentialing process exist?
2. If a credentialing process does exist, is it regulated by the state government, by the federal government, and/or a national professional association?
3. What are the degree requirements for being credentialed?
4. What post degree experiences are required for being credentialed?
5. Is a test required to become credentialed?

PART IV: MULTICULTURAL/ADVOCACY COMPETENCIES

XI. Multicultural Counseling Competencies

ACA's Multicultural Counseling Competencies provide the attitudes and beliefs, knowledge, and skills that students should have in three areas: (1) awareness of own cultural values and biases, (2) awareness of client's worldview, and (2) culturally appropriate intervention strategies (Roysircar, Arredondo, Fuertes, Ponterotto, & Toporek, 2003). Using Table 3.2 and cross-referencing the Multicultural Competencies provided in Appendix B, in the space provided, indicate in "a" if you need to be better trained in the area, "b" if you are somewhat trained in that area, or "c" if you are well-trained in that area. If you and your instructor desire, you may compare your results to others in class. For instance, if I believe I need to improve the attitudes and beliefs I have relative to gaining "cultural self-awareness and sensitivity to one's own cultural heritage..." (item I.A.1 in Appendix B), I would place an "a" in item 1 under attitudes and beliefs and across from Counselor Awareness of Own Cultural Values and Biases.

Table 3.2: Self-Assessment of Multicultural Competencies

	Attitudes and Beliefs	Knowledge	Skills
Counselor Awareness of Own Cultural Values and Biases	1. 2. 3. 4.	1. 2. 3.	1. 2.
Counselor Awareness of Client's Worldview	1. 2.	1. 2. 3.	1. 2.
Culturally Appropriate Intervention Strategies	1. 2. 3.	1. 2. 3. 4. 5..	1. 2. 3. 4. 5. 6. 7.

XII. Advocacy Competencies

The Advocacy Competencies encompass three areas (client/student, school/community, public arena), each of which are divided into two levels: whether the counselor is "acting on behalf" or "acting with" the competency area (see Figure 3.1). For instance, with the client competency, a counselor might "act with" a client to help the client identify strengths and resources in order to feel empowered and advocate for himself or herself; *or*, "on behalf" of the client, the counselor might assist the client in accessing needed services. The competencies run from the *microlevel* (focus on client) to the *macrolevel* (focus on system). Figure 3.1 shows the three competency areas, each divided into two levels. In Appendix C, the competencies are explained and examples of competency areas and levels are given.

Figure 3.1: ACA Advocacy Competencies

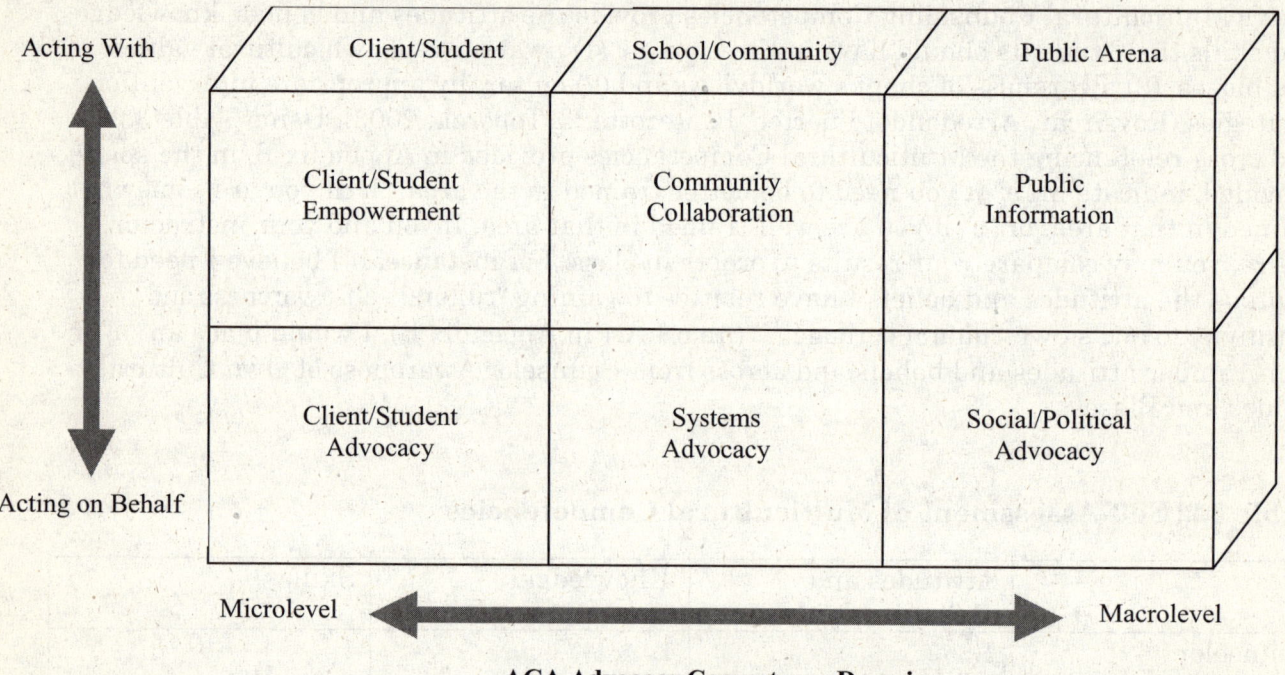

ACA Advocacy Competency Domains

Source: Toporek, R. L., & Lewis, J. A., & Crethar, H. C. (2009). Promoting systemic change through the ACA advocacy competencies. *Journal of Counseling and Development, 87,* p. 267.

6. Using the same scale used in Exercise XI, provide the letter that best describes your level of comfort in each of the six areas on the face of the cube (e.g., client/student empowerment, client/student advocacy, community collaboration, etc.). Write "a" if you need to be better trained in the area, "b" if you are somewhat trained, or "c" if you are well-trained. If you and your instructor desire, you may compare your results to others in class.

7. Some argue it is not the counselor's role to advocate "on behalf" of the client in the political arena. Write down your thoughts on this as well as positive and negative aspects of advocating for a client. Discuss in small groups.

XIII. Ethical and Professional Vignettes (The ACA's code is at www.counseling.org under "Resources"). In responding to the following, consider referring to the ACA's code.
1. After graduating, a fellow student in your CACREP-accredited counseling program takes and passes the National Counselor Exam (NCE). He then rents office space and advertises in the local newspaper saying, "Individual, Group, and Family Counseling by a Nationally Certified Counselor." Is this ethical? Is this professional? Is this legal in your state? Do the laws vary from state to state? Should you say anything to the student?
2. A rehabilitation counselor colleague of yours tells you he is interested in practicing as a family therapist. Is this ethical? Is this professional? Is this legal? Should you say anything to your colleague?
3. A colleague of yours runs into a former client at a social get-together. The client asks your colleague out, and the colleague accepts the offer after reflecting on the fact that the client has not been in counseling for the last five years. Is this ethical? Is this professional? Is this legal? Is this wise? Should you say anything to your colleague?
4. A licensed school counselor advertises in the local newspaper that she is facilitating a "parent-teen communication group." She facilitates the group on the weekends and has made an arrangement with her school where she can use space for a nominal fee. She charges $20 for each person in the group and keeps her profits. Is this ethical? Is this professional? Is this legal? Should you say anything to this colleague?
5. A licensed school counselor, who is not a licensed professional counselor, advertises that he is doing "short-term individual counseling." He does this part time at a local private practice clinic. Is this ethical? Is this professional? Is this legal? Should you say anything to him?
6. A colleague advertises that she is a licensed professional counselor candidate. She has completed all requirements for her license, but has not yet passed her licensure exam. She is doing private practice under supervision. How can the word "candidate" be misleading? Is this ethical? Is this professional? Is this legal?
7. You know that a friend of yours is practicing without a license. You tell a colleague who tells you that if you do not speak directly to your friend and/or report it, he will report you for not addressing an ethical violation. Is he acting ethically? Professionally? Are you in violation of the law? What should you do?
8. At the agency in which you work, you are counseling a number of clients who are adamantly "pro-life." You decide to attend a local "pro-choice" rally on the weekend. It is likely your clients will see your picture or name in the local newspaper. Are you acting ethically? Professionally? Is this a good choice to make?
9. A client you have been working with at your agency tells you she might harm her husband. You are concerned that her threats may be real. After leaving your office, you consult with your supervisor and decide to contact the husband. She sues you for breaking confidentiality. Have you acted ethically? Professionally? Have you acted within the law? Can your client sue you? If you have to go to court, what can you do to bolster your case?
10. As a private practitioner, you decide to not purchase malpractice insurance and take your chances. Are you acting ethically? Professionally? Are you acting within the law? Are you acting foolishly?
11. As a counselor in an agency, you decide to not purchase malpractice insurance and take your chances. Are you acting ethically? Professionally? Are you acting within the law? Are you acting foolishly?

12. As a school counselor, you decide to not purchase malpractice insurance and take your chances. Are you acting ethically? Professionally? Are you acting within the law? Are you acting foolishly?
13. A counselor you know has decided to try out a new technique involving extreme verbal confrontations of the client. You are familiar with the literature on client outcomes, and this technique does not seem to be in line with the research. Is he acting ethically? Professionally? Legally? What is your professional/ethical obligation?
14. As a counselor at a mental health center, you work daily with clients who are taking medications. One of your clients who has been taking Prozac continues to tell you that she is quite depressed. You say to her, "No problem, you need your medication changed, and I'll arrange that," and you refer her to the staff psychiatrist. Have you responded to the client in an ethical manner? Have you responded in a professional manner? Do you have other options?
15. You are personally opposed to the killing of animals for fur coats, and one of your clients walks in with a full-length new mink coat. She says to you, "Isn't this coat gorgeous?" at which point you respond by saying, "How many minks were killed to make that?" Have you responded ethically? Professionally? What should you do if your personal moral code interferes with you ethical guidelines?
16. The same person as in vignette 15 goes on to tell you that the minks that were raised for her coat came from an illegal mink ranch. In fact, you realize the treatment of the animals was probably horrible. Do you have any legal obligation to report this illegal ranch?
17. You are opposed to any kind of pornography. As the result of local community standards, the sale of any x-rated materials has been prohibited. Your client tells you that he is selling x-rated videos "underground" to the public within the local community. What is your moral responsibility? What is your ethical responsibility? What is your legal responsibility?
18. You have decided to forego licensure as a professional counselor, and instead of doing counseling you offer "educational workshops and periodic individual meetings." You advertise these as "coaching sessions" and state that you will offer "positive-goal-directed, short-term motivational sessions." Can you practice like this without a license? Is this counseling? Can you be sued for practicing without a license?
19. A client of yours who has been working on becoming more assertive with her spouse and at work finds out that she is being underpaid at work for the same services that other males in her position make. She asks you to write a letter for her, which she will sign, to send to her boss. Is this appropriate given the advocacy competencies? Are you working on "behalf" of your client? What implications might such an action have in your client's life?
20. Despite having little or no training in working with Ethiopian clients, you decide to take on, in family counseling, an Ethiopian family who has just moved to this country. Is this ethical? Is this professional? Is this wise? Should you work with these clients? What alternatives do you have?

CHAPTER 4

INDIVIDUAL APPROACHES TO COUNSELING

I: Your Theoretical Approach and Conceptual Orientation

The following scale offers you a way of determining to which theory of counseling and broad conceptual perspective you are most similar (a somewhat more user-friendly version can be found at http://www.odu.edu/~eneukrug/therapists/survey.html). To discover your theoretical and conceptual orientations, read each of the following items, and using the scale below, write in the spaces provided how strongly you feel about each item (write in a 1, 2, 3, 4, or 5). Then follow the directions for scoring found after the survey.

| I Don't Believe This | 1 | 2 | 3 | 4 | 5 | I Feel Extremely Certain |
| Statement at All | | | | | | This Statement Is True |

_____1. Instincts (e.g., hunger, thirst, survival, sex, and aggression) are very strong motivators of behavior.

_____2. Psychological symptoms represent a desire to regain repressed parts of ourselves as well as parts of the self that have never been revealed to consciousness.

_____3. Environmental influences on the child can lead to the development of a neurotic character, but through education and therapy, the person can change.

_____4. Children learn behaviors through conditioning (e.g., positive reinforcement, punishment).

_____5. We are born with the potential for rational or irrational thinking.

_____6. We are born with a predisposition toward certain disorders that could reveal themselves under stressful conditions.

_____7. We are born with five needs: survival, love and belonging, power, freedom, and fun.

_____8. We are born into a world that has no inherent meaning or purpose, and we subsequently create our own meaning and purpose.

_____9. An inborn actualizing tendency lends direction toward reaching our full potential.

_____10. We are born with the capacity to embrace an infinite number of personality dimensions.

_____11. Reality is created through interactions or discussions within one's social circle.

_____12. Change can occur in fewer than six sessions. Extended therapy is often detrimental.

_____13. Deciding how to satisfy instincts (e.g., hunger, thirst, survival, sex, and aggression) occurs mostly unconsciously.

_____14. Revealing unconscious material to consciousness allows for an integrated "whole" person.

_____15. We all are striving for perfection in our effort to be whole and complete.

_____16. Past and present conditioning make us who we are.

_____17. Irrational thinking leads to emotional distress, dysfunctional behaviors, and criticism of self and others.

_____18. By understanding one's cognitive processes (thinking), one can manage and change the way one lives.

_____19. We all have a quality world containing mental pictures of the people, things, and beliefs most important in meeting our unique needs.

_____20. We all struggle with the basic questions of what it is to be human.

_____21. Children continually assess whether interactions are positive or negative to their actualizing process, or way of living in the world.

_____22. The mind, body, and soul operate in unison; they cannot be separated.

_____23. Values held by those in power are disseminated through language and become the norms against which we compare ourselves.

_____24. Individuals can find exceptions to their problems and build on those exceptions to find new ways of living in the world.

_____25. Our personality is framed at a very young age and is quite difficult to change.

_____26. Primordial images that we all have interact with repressed material to create psychological complexes (e.g., mother complex; Peter Pan complex).

_____27. Children's experiences by age 5 years, and memories of those experiences, are critical factors in personality development.

_____28. Behaviors are generally conditioned and learned in very complex and subtle ways.

_____29. Although learning and biological factors influence the development of rational or irrational thinking, it is the individual who sustains his or her type of thinking.

_____30. Core beliefs (underlying beliefs that map our world) are the basis for a person's feelings, behaviors, and physiological responses.

_____31. We can only choose our actions and thoughts; our feelings and our physiology result from those choices.

_____32. We are born alone, will die alone, and except for periodic moments when we encounter another person deeply, we live alone.

_____33. The "self" has a need to be regarded positively by significant others.

_____34. From birth, the individual is in a constant state of self-regulation through a process of need identification and need fulfillment.

_____35. Psychopathology (mental disorders) is a social construction. There is no separate reality that supports its existence.

_____36. Although many therapies describe structures that affect functioning (e.g., id, ego, self-actualizing tendency), there is no objective reality proving their existence.

_____37. The development of defense mechanisms (repression, denial, projection) is a way of managing instincts.

_____38. Archetypes, or inherited unconscious primordial images, provide the psyche with its tendency to perceive the world in certain ways that we identify as human.

_____39. As children, how we learn to cope with inevitable feelings of inferiority affects our personality development.

_____40. Conditioning (e.g., positive reinforcement, punishment) can lead to a multitude of personality characteristics.

_____41. When our cognitive processes result in irrational thinking, we tend to have self-defeating emotions and exhibit dysfunctional behaviors.

_____42. Genetics, biological factors, and experiences combine to produce specific core beliefs that affect how we behave and feel.

_____43. At any point in one's life, one can evaluate one's behaviors, thoughts, feelings, and physiology, and make new choices that better meet one's needs.

_____44. Meaningfulness, as well as a limited sense of freedom, comes through consciousness and the choices we make.

_____ 45. Because they want to be loved, children will often act in a way in which significant others want them to act instead of acting in a manner that is real or congruent with themselves.

_____ 46. Parental dictates, social mores, and peer norms can prevent a person from attaining satisfaction of a need. This unsatisfied need can affect us in ways of which we are unaware.

_____ 47. Constant discourse and interactions with others within one's social milieu leads to the development of a sense of self.

_____ 48. Language endemic in culture, society, and the individual's social sphere determines the nature of reality.

_____ 49. Because we spend the majority of our time unconsciously struggling to satisfy our unmet needs, happiness is an elusive feeling experienced infrequently.

_____ 50. We are born with the mental functions of sensation/intuition and thinking/feeling, which affect our perceptions. Their relative strengths are affected by how we were raised.

_____ 51. At an early age, we develop a private logic that moves us toward dysfunctional behaviors or toward wholeness.

_____ 52. By carefully analyzing how behaviors are conditioned, one can understand why an individual exhibits his or her current behavioral repertoire.

_____ 53. Events do not cause negative emotions, but the belief about the events.

_____ 54. We all have automatic thoughts (fleeting thoughts about what we perceive and experience) that result in a set of behaviors, feelings, and physiological responses.

_____ 55. When language shows caring and the taking of responsibility, good choices are made. When language is blaming, critical, and judgmental, poor choices are made.

_____ 56. We sometimes avoid living authentically and experiencing life fully because we are afraid to look squarely at how we are making meaning in our lives.

_____ 57. Anxiety, and related symptoms, can be conceptualized as a signal to the individual that he or she is acting in a nongenuine way and not living fully.

_____ 58. Breaking free from defenses (e.g., repression) allows one to fully experience the present and live a saner life.

_____ 59. Reality is a social construction, and each person's reality is organized and maintained through his or her narrative and discourse with others.

_____ 60. Pathology, in all practical purposes, does not exist and is not inherently found within a person.

_____ 61. Early child-rearing practices are largely responsible for our personality development.

_____ 62. People are born with a tendency to be either extraverted (e.g., being outgoing) or introverted (e.g., being an observer, looking inward).

_____ 63. Child experiences, and the memories of them, impact each of the unique abilities and characteristics integral to the development of our character or personality.

_____ 64. By identifying what behaviors have been conditioned, one can eliminate undesirable behaviors and set goals to acquire more functional ways of acting.

_____ 65. The depth at which and length of time for which one experiences a self-defeating emotion is related to one's beliefs about an event, not to the event directly.

_____ 66. Automatic thoughts (fleeting thoughts about what we perceive) reinforce core beliefs we have about the world.

_____ 67. Needs can only be satisfied in the present, so focusing on how past needs were not met is useless.

____68. People can gain a personally meaningful and authentic existence by making new choices that involve facing life's struggles honestly and directly.
____69. Being around people who are real, empathic, and show positive regard results in the individual becoming more real.
____70. The ultimate way of living involves allowing oneself access to all of what is available to one's experience. Essentially, now = awareness = reality.
____71. Problems individuals have are a function of their problem-saturated stories or narratives. However, new preferred stories can be generated.
____72. Problems are the result of language passed down by families, culture, and society, and dialogues between people.

SCORING THE SURVEY

Scoring I: Psychodynamic Approaches. Place the numbers you chose across from the respective item. In each column, add up your score for each theory and divide the total by 30. That will give you the percentage score for that approach. Place your percentage in the parentheses. For the "psychodynamic score," add the total scores from each of the bottom rows and place it in the far right column. Divide that score by 90, and that will give you the percentage score for psychodynamic therapy. Place that percentage in the parentheses next to *psychodynamic*. This gives your overall score for this particularly conceptual orientation, which encompasses the theories listed.

Psychoanalysis( )	Analytical( )	Individual Psychology( )	Psychodynamic( )
1 ___	2 ___	3 ___	
13 ___	14 ___	15 ___	
25 ___	26 ___	27 ___	
37 ___	38 ___	39 ___	
49 ___	50 ___	51 ___	
61 ___	62 ___	63 ___	
Total: ___	___	___	___

Scoring II: Existential-Humanistic Approaches. Place the numbers you chose across from the respective item. In each column, add up your score for each theory and divide the total by 30. That will give you the percentage score for that approach. Place your percentage in the parentheses. For the "existential-humanistic score," add the total scores from each of the bottom rows and place it in the far right column. Divide that score by 90, and that will give you the percentage score for existential-humanistic therapy. Place that percentage in the parentheses next to *existential-humanistic*. This gives your overall score for this particularly conceptual orientation, which encompasses the theories listed.

Existential( )	Person-Centered( )	Gestalt( )	Existential-Humanistic( )
8 ___	9 ___	10 ___	
20 ___	21 ___	22 ___	
32 ___	33 ___	34 ___	
44 ___	45 ___	46 ___	
56 ___	57 ___	58 ___	
68 ___	69 ___	70 ___	
Total: ___	___	___	

Scoring III: Cognitive-Behavioral Approaches. Place the numbers you chose across from the respective item. In each column, add up your score for each theory and divide the total by 30. That will give you the percentage score for that approach. Place your percentage in the parentheses. For the "cognitive-behavioral score," add the total scores from each of the bottom rows and place it in the far right column. Divide that score by 120, and that will give you the percentage score for cognitive-behavioral therapy. Place that percentage in the parentheses next to *cognitive-behavioral*. This gives your overall score for this particularly conceptual orientation, which encompasses the theories listed.

Behavioral( )	Cognitive-REBT( )	Reality Behavioral( )	Cognitive–Therapy( )	Behavioral( )
4 ___	5 ___	6 ___	7 ___	
16 ___	17 ___	18 ___	19 ___	
28 ___	29 ___	30 ___	31 ___	
40 ___	41 ___	42 ___	43 ___	
52 ___	53 ___	54 ___	55 ___	
64 ___	65 ___	66 ___	67 ___	
Total: ___	___	___	___	___

Scoring IV: Post-Modern Approaches. Place the numbers you chose across from the respective item. In each column, add up your score for each theory and divide the total by 30. That will give you the percentage score for that approach. Place your percentage in the parentheses. For the "post-modern score," add the total scores from each of the bottom rows and place it in the far right column. Divide that score by 60, and that will give you the percentage score for post-modern therapy. Place that percentage in the parentheses next to *post-modern*. This gives your overall score for this particularly conceptual orientation, which encompasses the theories listed.

Narrative( )	Solution-Focused( )	Post-Modern( )
11 ___	12 ___	
23 ___	24 ___	
35 ___	36 ___	
47 ___	48 ___	
59 ___	60 ___	
71 ___	72 ___	
Total: ___	___	___

RESULTS

Your scores represent the percent of items you endorsed in each theoretical area as well as the percent of items you endorsed for the combined theories in a specific conceptual orientation (psychodynamic, existential-humanistic, cognitive-behavioral, and post-modern).

For descriptions of each of the theoretical approaches as well as the conceptual orientations in which you can find each of the approaches, see Appendix D.

II: Understanding Your View of Human Nature

For the four items that follow, circle *all* that describe your view of a person. Take all circled items and use them to write a paragraph describing your view of human nature. (Note how each statement represents a perspective on one's view of human nature).

1. *Innate at Birth.* I believe people are born
   a. good
   b. bad
   c. neutral
   d. with original sin
   e. restricted by their genetics
   f. with a growth force that allows them to change throughout life
   g. capable of being anything they want to be
   h. with sexual drives that consciously and unconsciously affect their lives
   i. with aggressive drives that consciously and unconsciously affect their lives
   j. with social drives that consciously and unconsciously affect their lives
   k. other attributes? _____

2. *The Developing Person.* Personality development is greatly influenced by
   a. genetics
   b. learning
   c. language
   d. drives
   e. biology
   f. environment
   g. relationships with others
   h. feelings of inferiority
   i. early child-rearing patterns
   j. modeling others' behaviors
   k. values taught to us
   l. developmental issues (e.g., puberty)
   m. conscious decisions
   n. the unconscious
   o. instincts
   p. cultural influences
   q. primordial images
   r. other_____

3. *The Change Process.* As people grow older, I believe they are
   a. capable of major changes in their personality
   b. capable of moderate changes in their personality
   c. capable of minor changes in their personality
   d. incapable of change in their personality
   e. determined by their early childhood experiences
   f. determined by their genetics
   g. determined by how they were conditioned and reinforced
   h. determined by unconscious motivations
   i. able to transcend or go beyond early childhood experiences

4. *The Focus of Change.* Change is likely to be most facilitated by a focus on
   a. the conscious mind
   b. the unconscious mind
   c. thoughts
   d. behaviors
   e. feelings
   f. early experiences
   g. the past
   h. the present
   i. the future
   j. the use of medications
   k. unfinished business
   l. repressed memories
   m. biology
   n. language
   o. memories
   p. one's "real" self
   q. other _____

III: Classification of Theoretical Approaches

Below are ways to classify major theories of counseling and therapy. First, make a list of theories you know (e.g., person-centered, psychoanalytic, Gestalt, reality therapy, cognitive therapy, etc.) (need help, go to http://enwikipediaorg/wiki/List_of_psychotherapies). Then, based on your knowledge, place each theory under the categories where you think it belongs. Keep in mind that a theory can be listed under different categories. When you have finished, form small groups and discuss your listings.

1) Existential | Cognitive | Behavioral | Psychodynamic
   _____ | _____ | _____ | _____
   _____ | _____ | _____ | _____
   _____ | _____ | _____ | _____

2) Self-Oriented | Other-Oriented | Socially-Oriented
   _____ | _____ | _____
   _____ | _____ | _____
   _____ | _____ | _____
   _____ | _____ | _____

3) Directive | Somewhat Directive | Nondirective
   _____ | _____ | _____
   _____ | _____ | _____
   _____ | _____ | _____
   _____ | _____ | _____

4) Strongly Confrontative | Somewhat Confrontative | Not Confrontative
   _____ | _____ | _____
   _____ | _____ | _____
   _____ | _____ | _____

5) Therapist-Centered | Collaborative | Client-Centered
   _____ | _____ | _____
   _____ | _____ | _____
   _____ | _____ | _____

6) Focus on Past | Focus on Present | Focus on Future
   _____ | _____ | _____
   _____ | _____ | _____
   _____ | _____ | _____

7) Brief Approach | Moderate Length | Long-Term Treatment
   _____ | _____ | _____
   _____ | _____ | _____
   _____ | _____ | _____

IV. Literature, Pop Psychology, and Theory

In groups of three or four, identify a "self-help" or "pop psych" book to critique. After reviewing the book, answer the following questions:
1. Does the work explicitly identify itself as being based on a theoretical framework?
2. If there is not a clear theoretical framework, can you identify the view of human nature from which the author's book is based?
3. Does the book show consistency in theory and/or view of human nature throughout? In other words, does the author seem to stay within his or her theoretical framework and/or view of human nature?
4. What specific points do you find intriguing in the book?
5. Do you think the work can be applied in your personal life? How?
6. Do you think the work can be applied in your professional life? How?
7. Do you see any possible negative impacts of the use of this book?

* This exercise was adapted from material by Dr. Thomas W. Blume, Oakland University. His contribution is greatly appreciated.

V. Name That Theory

In groups of three to five, conduct 10-minute mock individual counseling sessions. Each student will be assigned the following roles:

Client: Present a real-life problem to the counselor. Be cautious of divulging sensitive information or material you may not want others to know about.

Counselor: Utilize a counseling theory of your choice; however, do not disclose the approach to the client or observer(s).

Observer(s): Take note of the strategies and techniques utilized in the mock counseling session and when the role-play is complete.

When you are finished, as a group, discuss the following:
1. What theoretical approach do the observers and the client believe were implemented? Are you correct?
2. What techniques were identified?
3. Were the techniques consistent with the theoretical approach?
4. Does the theoretical approach make sense with the presenting problem of the client?
5. Did the client feel as if the theoretical approach taken was reasonable for his or her presenting problem?
6. What other techniques or strategies from the theoretical approach could have been used?
7. Would other theoretical approach(es) could have been used with this client?

If time allows, students can switch roles and do another role-play.

* This exercise was adapted from material by Dr. Jeffrey Warren, North Carolina State University. His contribution is greatly appreciated.

VI: Differing Theoretical Orientations as Applied to Clients

With the following clients, think about how varying theoretical orientations would be applied to their situations. Specifically, how would the theory explain the client's current predicament, and how would it be used to help the client change? Your instructor may wish to assign students to various groups, which would describe how the different theories might work with the clients below.

A. The Story of Jill

Jill is a 32-year-old married mother of two children, aged seven and two. She states that prior to getting married six years ago, she drank a lot and smoked pot daily. She notes that at that time in her life, she used to "hang out with bikers and sleep with a lot of guys." She has "settled down" since then, but she reports that recently she started hanging out with her neighbor Steven, drinking again, and is thinking about having an affair with him. She states that she loves her husband, but he has not been paying attention to her lately. She describes her husband as "a real nice guy who never talks about his feelings." She is pleased that he does not drink much or do drugs. Although she maintained "average" grades in high school, she never completed school and would like to eventually obtain her GED. She notes that she works part time in a factory. She reports having frequent anxiety attacks and rarely leaves her house other than to go to work.

Jill is the second child in a family of four and states that while growing up, her father was verbally abusive, drank a lot, and generally didn't pay attention to her. She reports that since he stopped drinking a few years ago, he has become closer to her. She describes her mother as being "nice but shy," and wished when she was young that her mother had stood up to her father's constant drinking and verbal abuse. She experienced her childhood as chaotic because she never knew if her father would blow up at her or other members of her family when he was drunk. Jill reports that she admires her brother, who is two years older than she, because he has "kept his job, loves his wife, and has kept clean." Her sisters, who are two and four years younger than she, are single, dropped out of school, involved with the "wrong crowd," and into drugs. No one in her family has ever received a high school diploma.

B. The Story of Harley

Harley was recently released from the state mental hospital where he has spent most of his adolescence. He has had acute schizophrenic episodes since he was 13 years old. His parents abandoned him when he was nine, at which point he went to live with an aunt and uncle. After living with them for four years, he began to have auditory and visual hallucinations. He also, at this point, accused them of having sexually abused him. He was hospitalized in the state mental institution for schizophrenia and spent the next five years in and out of the state hospital and various foster homes. Harley just turned 18.

Harley is currently taking anti-psychotic and anti-anxiety medications and is in the day treatment program at the local community mental health center. At day treatment, he spends the day in support groups, doing vocational skills training, and socializing. He has few memories of his childhood, but what he can remember is very painful. For instance, he has vague memories of his parents being physically abusive, and memories of being sexually abused by his uncle while his aunt stood by. Harley's lifelong dream is to own a motorcycle, and he seems to talk about motorcycles as if they are his lover. Confidentially, he reports having had sexual feelings toward a motorcycle. Harley has few friends and has an impulsive temper; that is, he periodically just blows up. Although he generally does not act out physically toward people, on rare occasions he has been known to attack someone in an impulsive rage. His medication seems to help him with his outbursts.

C. The Story of Joshua

Joshua is 12 years old and in seventh grade. He is the youngest of three children, having two older sisters, 14 and 15. Joshua has always done well in school and was placed in the gifted program. During the first part of the school year, Joshua obtained As, but after the winter break, his grades drastically dropped to Cs and Ds. He seems comfortable at school socially and does not report using drugs. He seems to hang out with some good kids. He has recently entered puberty, and he secretly reports to you that he is feeling very "horny" all of the time. However, he adamantly states that this has not affected his studying habits. He reports feeling "a little depressed," and he seems anxious while talking with you. He is constantly looking around and doesn't seem able to focus. He notes, "My parents aren't arguing any more than usual."

When consulting with Joshua's parents, it becomes obvious that his father is severely depressed, while his mother admits to being bulimic, "throwing up a few times a day." They have little if any sexual relationship, and seem to talk about Joshua's problems whenever they are asked about themselves. They admit that their relationship is "not what it used to be." Joshua's two older sisters are doing well in school and report no problems. Neither sister understands why everyone is making such a big deal over Joshua. His 14-year-old sister says, "He is just a jerk. I'm surprised he's done as well as he has." His oldest sister says, "I would have problems if mom and dad doted over me like they do over him."

VII: The Implementation of Varying Theoretical Approaches

Describe how each of the key therapeutic elements listed in Table 4.1 could be applied in the settings listed (see example listed).

Table 4.1: Key Therapeutic Elements

	Length of Treatment	Focus on Consciousness or Unconsciousness	Focus on Feelings	Focus on Actions	Focus on Cognitions	Development Focus
Elementary School Counselor	Brief treatment: not enough time for long-term counseling. Refer out for long-term treatment.	Focus on consciousness, as unconsciousness requires long-term treatment. Help students identify conscious thoughts to recognize the relationship between consciousness and actions.	Help students identify feelings, talk about them, and make sense out of them. Use aids (e.g., feeling charts, play therapy) to help students identify feelings.	Help students identify specific action plans to address problem areas.	Teach students the basics of "self-talk." Show them how what one thinks can affect one's feelings and behaviors.	Identify developmental stages (e.g., Erikson's Industry vs. Inferiority) and make appropriate preventive workshops for students.
Middle School Counselor						
High School Counselor						
Mental Health Center Counselor						
College Counselor						
Rehabilitation Counselor						
Private Practitioner						
Crisis Counselor						

TABLE 4.1 (Cont'd): Key Therapeutic Elements

	Focus on Past	Focus on Present	Focus on Future	Focus on Systemic Issues (e.g., family, community society)	Focus on Relationships
Elementary School Counselor	Discuss past to identify treatment strategies, but don't harbor on them due to time limits.	Focus on present-day activities and behaviors that can help change the student.	Develop long-term attainable goals.	Understand family, community, and societal impact on child. Foster and advocate for systemic change.	Determine what relationships impact a child and make strategies for change (e.g., peer, family, teacher).
Middle School Counselor					
High School Counselor					
Mental Health Center Outpatient Therapist					
College Counselor					
Rehabilitation Counselor					
Private Practitioner					
Crisis Counselor					

VIII. Using Cinema to Teach Counseling Theory

Films can often illustrate major points of many different theoretical orientations. Using the list of films below, or others of your choosing with your instructor's approval, view and then discuss how each of the movies may amplify different points from varying theoretical orientations.

1. *The Diary of Anne Frank* (1959) and *I Heart Huckabees* (2004) for existential therapy.
2. *My Fair Lady (2964), Tea with Mussolini* (1999), and *Firefly Dreams* (2001) for Adlerian therapy.
3. *Drugstore Cowboy* (1989), *What About Bob* (1991), and *Dead Man Walking* (1995) for cognitive-behavioral approaches.
4. *Breaking the Waves* (1997) and the *Star Wars* series for Jungian concepts.
5. *Portnoy's Complaint* (1972) and *The Human Stain* (2003) for psychoanalytic concepts.
6. *Ordinary People* (1980) and *Good Will Hunting* (1997) for an eclectic approach.
7. *The Matrix* (1999), *A Beautiful Mind* (2001), and *Inception* (2010) for post-modern movies.

IX: Adapting Theories to Brief and Solution-Focused Approaches

After examining some of the theories from your text, discuss how they might be applied in a brief treatment approach. Specifically, for each theory:

1. Explain its view of human nature from a brief treatment focus
2. Adapt the therapeutic relationship to a brief therapy approach
3. Apply its major goals to a brief therapy modality
4. Apply the techniques to a brief therapy modality

X. Disadvantages/Advantages of Brief and Solution-Focused Approaches

After reviewing your response to Exercise IX, list the advantages and disadvantages to adapting a brief approach to the various theories.

XI: Eclecticism or Theoretical Integration

A. Understanding Our View of Human Nature

Today, many counselors use an integrative approach when working with clients. Such an approach is not a "hodge podge" of techniques from different theories, but a well thought out theoretical approach that integrates, in a meaningful fashion, concepts and techniques from different theories. To develop such an approach, one must first have a clear understanding of his or her view of human nature. Table 4.2 is designed to help you do this. For each approach listed, pick out 1 to 4 key concepts that you think are important and list them in the table. An example of some key concepts I believe are important from each theory is listed in Table 4.2. Then, go on to Exercise B.

B. Determining Techniques Based on Our View of Human Nature

Using the items you picked in Table 4.2, write a paragraph or two about your integrative approach—or how you pull together all of the concepts you believe are important into one way of working with clients. The paragraph that follows is an example of one that I wrote using the words and terms in Table 4.2. The words and terms are italicized.

Table 4.2   **Theoretical Approach**

Approach	Concepts You Believe Are Critical			
Psychoanalysis	Early Child-Rearing	Unconscious		
Jungian Analysis	Complexes			
Individual Psychology	Memories			
Existential Therapy	Choice	The Relationship	Change	Journey
Gestalt Therapy	Figure-Ground			
Person-Centered Counseling	Empathy	Unconditional Positive Regard	Congruence	
Behavior Therapy	Reinforcement Contingences	Modeling		
Rational Emotive Behavior Therapy	Thinking Leads to Dysfunctional Behavior	Challenging One's Belief System		
Beck's Cognitive Therapy	Core Beliefs			
Reality Therapy	Seven Deadly Habits	Seven Caring Habits	Internal Control	
Narrative Therapy	Language	Cultural Milieu Constructs One's Sense of the World		
Solution-Focused Therapy	Respectful Curiosity	Looking at Solutions, Not Problems		

Sample Paragraph

I believe that a person is molded by others in his or her life through *language*, *modeling*, and *reinforcement contingencies*, which are a particular function of the *cultural milieu* in which one grew up. Although I believe that one's personality is molded most powerfully in *early childhood*, I also believe that one can *change* at any time throughout one's life if he or she can come to realize how his or her *conscious* and *unconscious* minds have impacted the kinds of *choices* he or she has made. A client can come to realize this impact if he or she is provided with a safe atmosphere to share thoughts with a counselor. Such an atmosphere is provided by a counselor showing a *respectful curiosity* about the client's predicament, and when a counselor is *empathic*, shows *unconditional positive regard*, and is *congruent*. In this environment, issues that were in the background and have been *unconscious* can slowly come into the *foreground* and into *consciousness*. As the counselor builds a *relationship* with the client, the client will slowly feel comfortable enough to begin the difficult *journey* of working on his or her issues, which have sometimes formed *complexes* or certain particular ways of being that are dysfunctional. As the client begins to see his or her issues more clearly, the counselor can help the client look at how embedded *core beliefs* continue dysfunctional behaviors. Slowly, clients can *challenge* their belief system, and new behaviors can be adopted. As the client realizes that he or she has *internal control* over his or her thinking, the client can increasingly focus on *solutions* rather than focusing on past problems. Over time, *change* will take place, and the client will adopt more effective ways of being with self and with others. Some of this will be demonstrated by the client giving up *seven deadly habits* and adopting the *seven caring habits*.

XI. Ethical, Legal, and Professional Vignettes

(The ACA's code is at www.counseling.org under "Resources"). In responding to the following, consider referring to the ACA's code.

A. Refer to Harley, Jill, and Joshua (Boxes 4.1, 4.2, and 4.3) to Discuss the Following Vignette.

1. While helping Jill find study classes for the GED exam, she reveals that sometimes when she's drinking she takes the belt out and "whacks my kids good because they just won't shut up." Do you break confidentiality and tell Child Protective Services? What are your ethical and legal obligations?

2. While driving to work one day, your car breaks down. Harley sees you and says, "I'm good with mechanical things, let me help for a small fee, besides I could use a little money for buying my bike." You want to get your car fixed, and you want Harley to have his bike. Do you let him help you? Is this considered a "dual" or "multiple" relationship?

3. One day, Jill tells you she is pregnant by Steven. She's going to have an abortion. Your state has a law requiring women to tell their spouses if they're to have an abortion. She refuses. What do you do? What are your ethical and legal obligations?

4. Jill's husband shows up at your office demanding information about his wife. You tell him that information obtained in counseling is confidential. He tells you that he'll sue you and the rest of this "fleabag" operation. What are your ethical and legal obligations?

5. You've been encouraging Jill for months to get involved in more social activities and to get out of the house more. One day, Jill unexpectedly shows up at your art class saying that she signed up for the same class. What do you do?

6. Jill tells you that from time to time, usually when she's drinking, she gets severely depressed and thinks about killing herself. You ask her if she has a plan, and she says, "Well, sometimes I think about just doing it with that gun my husband has." One day, she calls you; she's been drinking, and she tells you she's depressed. She hangs up, saying, "I don't know what I might do." What do you do?

7. Harley stops taking his medication, drops by your office, and seems pretty angry. He says, "That cheating Harley-Davidson dealer, he's trying to rip me off. He told me I

could have that bike at a discount and went back on his word." You try to talk with Harley, but he storms out of your office, saying, "I'm gonna get that man!" What do you do?

8. You decide to see Joshua's mother in a session by herself. During the session, she begins to tell you how attracted she is to you. How do you handle the situation? Do you reveal what she said to her husband? What if Joshua's father comes on to you instead? Does how you react make a difference if the person who comes on to you is of the same sex?

9. You discover that Joshua's mother is throwing up so often that her health may be at risk. She refuses to attend to this medical situation. What responsibility do you have to her? Must you break confidentiality and attempt to have her committed against her will to a psychiatric unit?

10. If you were told that you had a maximum of 10 sessions to work with Harley, Jill, or Joshua, how would you proceed? What is your ethical obligation for the proper treatment of the client? What if you believe that 10 sessions is not enough to do much good?

B. Other Vignettes

11. A psychologist colleague of yours encourages you to practice "Millennium Therapy," an intensive new therapeutic approach for which she has been trained and that, she says, has shown promising results with a vast array of clients. She says to you that she will offer you periodic, informal supervision, and encourages you to go to a local workshop on the technique. Should you follow through with this suggestion?

12. You are seeing a client who has struggled with moderate depression most of her life. You believe that you can only be effective with her in a long-term treatment regime; however, the HMO to which the client belongs only pays for brief treatment. You decide to see her for short-term counseling, get her on a medication regime to stabilize her, and encourage her to come back in six months. Have you acted ethically? Professionally? Legally?

13. A colleague of yours tells you she is eclectic in her approach. However, when she explains what she does, it is apparent that she is constantly adapting her view of human nature and changing her techniques to fit her client's current issues. In fact, with any one client, she changes her treatment approach on a weekly basis. Is what she is doing efficacious? Should you approach her and/or report her to an ethics committee?

14. A colleague of yours tells you he is conducting psychoanalysis with a client who has an obsessive-compulsive disorder. You know that he has little training in psychoanalysis and that psychoanalytic treatment of obsessive-compulsive disorder has not been shown to be effective. What should you do?

CHAPTER 5

COUNSELING SKILLS

I. The Office Environment
A. Creating Your Office
Take the furniture from Figure 5.1 and arrange it on a large piece of blank paper, creating your own office the way you would like it to be. Feel free to add your own furniture or to not use mine (excuse my taste in furniture!). Compare your office to the office of other students. What makes your office more or less conducive to the counseling relationship? Come up with a justification for your office arrangement based on your counseling style.

Figure 5.1

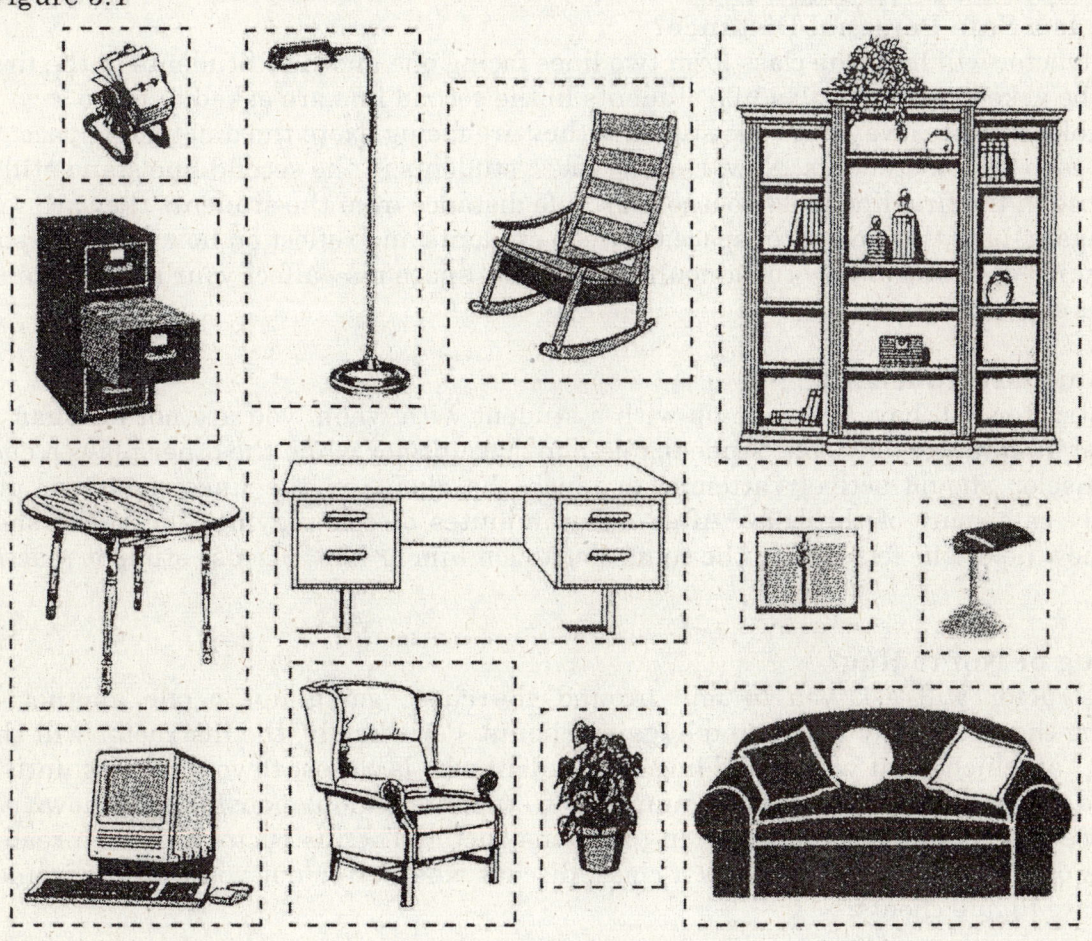

B. What Makes an Offensive Office?

Review the items below and reflect on whether or not you think any of them would be offensive to you or to potential clients if they came to your office. How does one balance one's own values and tastes relative to clients' values and taste?

- Feminist literature
- A bear rug
- Gay literature
- A cluttered desk
- Information on abortion
- A leather chair
- Fundamentalist religious literature
- A compulsively clean desk
- An AIDS pin
- A desk between you and your client
- Information on female and male sexuality
- A brochure supporting a politician

With your fellow students, discuss these items and others you might think are controversial.

II. Nonverbal Behavior and Touch

A. What Is a Safe Personal Distance?

Your instructor will have the class form two lines facing one another. Students in the first line will be asked to stand still while students in the second line are asked to move a comfortable distance away from the students they are facing. Note the amount of space between each pair of students. Now, reverse roles; students in the second line stand still while those in the first line move to a comfortable distance from the students they are facing. Again, note the amount of space between students and reflect on how much personal space you need. Consider how the amount of personal space may affect your relationship with your clients.

B. Do You Dare Touch Me?

Your instructor will have you pair up with a student with whom you are not familiar. For about 5 or 10 minutes, have one student role-play a counselor while the other plays a client. The counselor should actively attempt to touch the client on the knee, hand, or other (relatively safe) part of the body. After a few minutes of role-playing, the client should discuss how he or she felt having the counselor touch him or her. Discuss student reactions in class.

C. To Hug or Not to Hug?

Your instructor will ask you to mill around the class, going up to one another and discussing the ethics of touching and hugging clients. Periodically, the instructor will shout out "hug," at which point you should hug the student who is closest to you. Do this until you have had the opportunity to hug a number of students. Anonymously write down your experience of the exercise and pass it in to the instructor. The instructor will then read the reactions of students in the class. As a class, discuss whether or not you think it would be appropriate to hug clients.

D. Identifying Nonverbal Behavior

The following is a list of nonverbal behaviors that might occur in a counseling session. For each behavior, identify what you believe its meaning could be and how you might respond to the behavior.

1. A client nods his or her head
2. A client folds his or her arms
3. A client yawns
4. A client turns away from you
5. A client stops talking and becomes quiet
6. A client comes to the counseling session late
7. A client does not make eye contact
8. A client leans back
9. A client crosses his or her leg
10. A client starts to cry

* This exercise was adapted by Dr. Darrick Tovar-Murray, DePaul University. His contribution is greatly appreciated.

III: Listening Quiz

Take the listening quiz that follows. Place an X in the appropriate space to represent how you *generally* respond to someone when you are listening. Then, go through the quiz again, this time placing an O to represent how you think you *should* listen to another.

USUALLY	SOMETIMES	RARELY	
____	____	____	1. I try to determine what should be talked about during the interview.
____	____	____	2. When listening to someone, I prepare myself physically by sitting in a way that I can make sure that I hear what is being said.
____	____	____	3. I try to be "in charge" and lead the conversation.
____	____	____	4. I usually clear my mind and take on a nonjudgmental attitude when listening to another.
____	____	____	5. When listening to another, I try to tell the other my opinion of what he or she is doing.
____	____	____	6. I try to decide from the other's *appearance* whether or not what he or she is saying is worthwhile.
____	____	____	7. I attempt to ask questions if I need further clarification.
____	____	____	8. I try to judge from the person's opening statement whether or not I know what is going to be said.
____	____	____	9. I try to listen intently to feelings.
____	____	____	10. I try to listen intently to content.
____	____	____	11. I try to tell the other person what is "right" about what he or she is saying.
____	____	____	12. I try to "analyze" the situation and give interpretations.
____	____	____	13. I try to use *my* experiences to best understand the other person's feelings.
____	____	____	14. I try to convince the other person of the "correct" way to view the situation.
____	____	____	15. I try to have the last word.

After finishing the listening quiz, as a small group or as a class, define the term *listening*. You may want to use the definition below in developing your group definition. After you have defined the word *listening*, see if the answers you gave on your quiz reflect this definition. The *Oxford English Dictionary* asserts that "to listen" means 1) to hear attentively, 2) to give ear to, and 3) to pay attention to.

IV. Hindrances to Effective Listening

Break into triads and have each student take the number 1, 2, or 3. Next, your instructor will assign all number 1s and 2s to one of the topics below, with number 1 being "pro" the situation and number 2 being "con" the situation. Number 1 should role-play "pro" this situation, even if he or she is personally against the situation, and number 2 should role-play "con" this situation, even though he or she may personally be for this situation. After each person is finished stating a point of view, the other person should repeat back *verbatim* what he or she heard (e.g., number 1 talks, and number 2 repeats back verbatim what he or she heard). Note: this is repeating back verbatim, and *not* "reflective listening." Then number 2 talks, and number 1 repeats back verbatim what he or she heard. Take turns listening and repeating back verbatim what the other has said until your instructor tells you to stop. It is important to not tell the other person (verbally or nonverbally!) whether you are *actually* pro or con the situation. Not revealing your beliefs about the situation is good practice, as counselors often withhold their beliefs about particular subjects from clients. In fact, try never to tell other students what your true beliefs are!

Number 3s, you are to offer feedback about accuracy, help the other two people when they forget responses, and give feedback regarding body language. When the first situation is finished, your instructor will have numbers 2 and 3 do the second situation (2 be pro, 3 be con), and when that situation is finished, numbers 3 and 1 do the third situation (3 be pro, 1 be con). The non-participant is always the helper. When you have finished, the instructor will ask you to provide examples of ways in which you did not hear the other person. List these "hindrances to listening" on the board. Make sure you discuss some of the following hindrances: preoccupation, defensiveness, emotional blocks, and distractions.

Some Possible Situations: Abortion, capital punishment, torture of suspected terrorists, affirmative action, deficit spending, other?

V. Avoiding Counseling Clichés

As a group, your instructor will ask you to identify counseling responses that are clichés and write them on the board (e.g., "What was your mother like?" "I hearing you saying...," "So tell me more about that...," What did that feel like?" "Do you think this is due to your childhood?" and so forth). Then, break up into groups of 3 to 5 people, and have one person be a counselor, one a client, and the rest observers. Next, hand each student five clothespins and an index card. Each time the counselor uses one of the counseling clichés (or others perhaps not earlier identified), one of the observers should take a clothespin away and write the cliché on the index card. Continue the role-play for 10 to 15 minutes or until all the clothes pins are taken. At the end of the role-play, give the index card to the counselor for feedback. Have others do a similar role-play. Consider the following:
1. What are some of the positive and negative aspects of some of the clichés used?
2. As an inexperienced counselor, how can the use of clichés be helpful?
3. As an inexperienced counselor, how can the use of clichés be harmful?
4. How do you think clichés are used by experienced counselors?
5. How do you think your counseling style will change as you adapt new skills?

* This exercise was adapted from material by Angela Shores, doctoral candidate at North Carolina State University. Her contribution is greatly appreciated.

VI. Minimal Encouragers (Words, Phrases, and/or Gestures)

Minimal encouragers refer to words, phrases, and/or gestures that show a client that you are listening to him or her and encourage a client to talk about his or her reason for seeking counseling. Below are some examples:

Word	Phrase	Gesture
Okay	Keep going	Nodding
Uh-huh	Tell me more	Head shaking
Yes	Right, right, okay	Pause
Sure	I'm understanding you	Silent
Good	I hear you	Head nod
Right	That makes sense	Encouraging facial expression
Interesting	Good, good, good	Open hand gesture
Oh	I feel you	Eye contact
Hmmm	I sense that	Leaning forward
Continue	Please say more	Rubbing hands on chin

Divide in dyads and begin a counseling interview for 10 minutes. Make as many minimal encouragers as possible. Once you are done with the interview, answer the following questions:

1. What was it like to listen to another person?
2. What impact did minimal encourager(s) have on your ability to listen?
3. How many different types of minimal encouragers did you use?
4. What impact did minimal encourager(s) have on the person you interviewed?
5. Which minimal encouragers did you find useful and why?
6. Which minimal encouragers did you not find useful and why?

* This exercise was adapted by material from Dr. Darrick Tovar-Murray, DePaul University. His contribution is greatly appreciated.

VII. Making Empathic Responses

Empathy has been shown to be one of the most important counselor responses related to positive client outcomes. A good empathic response accurately reflects back to the client the feelings and the meaning of what the client has said. For the following situations, in the spaces provided, write the feeling followed by the meaning of what the client said. Then, write a statement that reflects back the feeling and meaning of the client, but this time in your own words. Share some of your responses in class and receive feedback from others about the accuracy of what you wrote.

Example: Distraught Wife to Counselor

Client: *My husband's such a do-nothing idiot. Since he lost his job, he just sits around all day like a log—he doesn't look for a job, doesn't cook, just does nothing.*

Counselor: *You feel <u>angry</u> because <u>your husband just sits around and doesn't do anything all day long</u>.* [Notice that this "formula response" has the feeling word "angry" followed by the content "your husband doesn't do anything all day long." Next, look at the example below which is a more "natural response" to the same client's predicament.]

Counselor: *I guess I hear how angry and disappointed you are over your husband not taking charge of his life.*

Now, respond to the following scenarios.

1. Teenager to Counselor
Client: *Why should I use condoms? I'm not going to get AIDS or nothing like that. Only fags get AIDS. Don't you think?*

Formula Response: _____

_____.

Natural Response: _____

_____.

2. Abused Wife to Counselor
Client: *I shake when I think of going back to him. He just keeps beating on me. But I don't know where else to go.*

Formula Response: _____

_____.

Natural Response: _____

_____.

3. Pregnant Teenager to Counselor
Client: *I hate my parents for wanting me to have an abortion. I want this baby, and I can bring it up myself. I'll quit school and get a job and bring the baby to work with me.*

Formula Response: _____

_____.

Natural Response: _____

_____.

4. Disabled Enlisted Person to Counselor
Client: *Even though I lost my leg, I have lots to live for. I have a good family, and I know I'm employable. I just hope I can get through rehab quickly.*

Formula Response: _____

_____.

Natural Response: _____

_____.

5. Older Person to Counselor
   Client: *Since I moved to this retirement home, I have nothing to live for. I can't drive anymore, and I know nobody here.*

Formula Response: _____
_____.

Natural Response: _____
_____.

6. Minority to Counselor
   Client: *I'm getting the shaft with my realtor. I keep telling her I want to move to this one community, and she can't find anything for sale there. I don't believe it!*

Formula Response: _____
_____.

Natural Response: _____
_____.

7. Pro-Life Person to Counselor
   Client: *Babies are dying! I'll do anything to close down those murdering abortion clinics.*

Formula Response: _____
_____.

Natural Response: _____
_____.

8. Pro-Choice Person to Counselor
   Client: *A woman has a right to choose what to do with her body, and I'm sick and tired of these pro-lifers interfering with other people's right to choose!*

Formula Response: _____
_____.

Natural Response: _____
_____.

9. Estranged Lover to Counselor
   Client: *So I wasn't faithful to my lover. So what! I loved him. He didn't have to leave me. I still was good to him despite my failings. I miss him so much!*

Formula Response: _____
_____.

Natural Response: _____
_____.

10. Estranged Wife to Counselor

Client: *I loved my husband, but I couldn't put up with his unfaithfulness any longer. He just couldn't give me the love I needed in a relationship. I'm sorry he is so depressed now, but I can't go back to him.*

Formula Response: _____
_____.

Natural Response: _____
_____.

VIII. Advanced Empathy

Sometimes, a counselor can make a response that goes deeper than what the client is stating he or she feels or understands about a situation. When the counselor senses deeper feelings and reflects those back, or when based on the client's statements the counselor can help the client *reframe* how he or she is viewing the situation, the counselor has made an advanced empathic response. For example, in the example at the beginning of Exercise VII, a counselor may say something like this:

Counselor: *Your life, particularly your marriage, has not turned out the way you had dreamed—I can see your disappointment.*

Other times, a counselor might use an analogy, metaphor, or visual image to bring forth deeper meanings to the client. For instance, in the same situation as above, the counselor might say this:

Counselor: *I have this image of you sitting on the floor in the middle of your living room. There is no furniture around you, and you're sobbing. Your husband is sitting on the floor in a corner, helpless, not knowing what to do.*

Now, using the same 10 scenarios as in Exercise VII, try to make an advanced empathic response to each client's predicament.

IX. Silence Is Golden

Break up into dyads and have one person role-play a counselor and the other a client. At an appropriate time, wait 30 seconds before you respond to the client. At another time, wait 20 seconds, then 10 seconds.
1. How did it feel to maintain silence for the specified periods?
2. Did your client break the silence by talking?
3. What might be some of the advantages and disadvantages of maintaining silence?
4. Do you think you could maintain silence for 30 seconds? 20 seconds? 10 seconds?

X. Basic Questions
A. Open vs. Closed, Direct vs. Indirect Questions

Your instructor will have you get into groups of six students. Have two students sit in the middle of the group, one role-playing a counselor, the other a client. Have the counselor intentionally ask as many different kinds of questions as possible and reasonable within a 10-minute role-play. Each student sitting on the outside of the circle should take turns writing down the questions asked. When you are finished, in small groups, determine if the questions are open or closed, direct or indirect, and place them accordingly into the grid located at the end of this exercise. Then, review the various quadrants and discuss the effectiveness of the various questions.

	Open	Closed
Direct		
Indirect		

B. Probing vs. Non-Probing, Confrontational vs. Non-Confrontational Questions

Using a grid like the one in "A," this time place some of the questions from the class activity into probing vs. non-probing, and confrontational vs. non-confrontational quadrants. As with Exercise A, discuss the efficacy of the various types of questions.

	Probing	Non-Probing
Confrontational		
Non-Confrontational		

XI. Solution-Focused Questions

Questions used by narrative and solution-focused counselors tend to look for times when individuals have coped effectively with a problem as well as exceptions to the problem. Such questions help clients believe that they can cope and offer hope for finding solutions rather than focusing on the problem. Below are some samples of coping questions, exception-seeking questions, and an example of the "miracle question," which has become popularized by the solution-focused approach. In groups of three, have two students role-play a counselor and client with the counselor practicing these kinds of questions. Either record the role-play or have the third person write down the questions asked. The third person can also be an objective evaluator of the process. When you are finished, discuss the efficacy of the questions used. Switch roles so every person in the triad gets to play the counselor.

Coping Questions
- What ways have you found to help manage or alleviate your _____ (e.g., depression, anxiety, anger, eating issues, etc.)?
- What other ways have you tried that were successful in alleviating your _____?
- I know you had trouble getting out of bed this morning because you were so _____. Can you tell me what enabled you to get yourself up?
- Your _____ seems to have impacted your eating, and you've lost some weight. How is it that you are sometimes able to eat a reasonable amount?

Exception-Seeking Questions
- I bet there have been times in your life when you have not felt _____ (e.g., depressed, anxiety, anger, eating issues, etc.)? Can you describe them for me?
- What was going on in your life when you did not feel _____?
- When undergoing hardships, people often have moments when they feel good. Can you describe times like that for me? What is going on with you during those times?

The Miracle Question
- Suppose a miracle happened while you were sleeping and the problem that brought you here was solved. What would your life look like? How would things be different?

XII. Self-Disclosure
Discuss the scenarios below relative to whether or not you believe self-disclosure would be appropriate.
1. A counselor shares with a new client, who is bulimic, that he too has struggled with an eating disorder and is now in recovery.
2. In a moment of deep sharing by a client, a counselor tells the client *she* cares about *her*.
3. In a moment of deep sharing by a client, a counselor tells the client *she* cares about *him*.
4. In a moment of deep sharing by a client, a counselor tells the client *he* cares about *her*.
5. In a moment of deep sharing by a client, a counselor tells the client *he* cares about *him*.
6. A counselor, who normally does not share personal issues with his client, tells a client he is in therapy for depression. He tells his client this in an effort to "normalize" counseling for the client.
7. With no intent to act on her feelings, a counselor tells her client she is attracted to him. She hopes the disclosure will model openness during the session.
8. With no intent to act on his feelings, a gay counselor tells his heterosexual male client he is attracted to him. The intent is to model openness and help the client work through his homophobic feelings. What if the client was gay?
9. A counselor shares with his client that he is a runner. He hopes that this disclosure will assist him in building his relationship with the client, who is also a runner.
10. A counselor shares with his client intimate issues about his extended family in hopes that the client will be more open in talking about his extended family.
11. A counselor shares with her client that she often gets into arguments with her husband, and later they "process" what has occurred. She does not offer particulars about the arguments, but hopes to instill the importance of the client processing issues with her partner.
12. Other _____.

XIII. Inadvertent and Intentional Modeling
In the literature, two types of modeling have generally been identified. *Inadvertent* modeling is when the counselor does *not* purposefully set out to change client behaviors. However, behavior change does occur as the client takes in the "being" of the counselor. For instance, the person-centered counselor is continually modeling the use of empathy. *Intentional* modeling, on the other hand, purposely models targeted behaviors in one of

three ways: (1) through the deliberate display of specific behaviors on the part of the helper (e.g., expressing empathy, being nonjudgmental, being assertive), (2) through the use of role-playing during the session (e.g., the counselor might role-play job interviewing techniques for the client), and (3) by teaching the client about modeling and encouraging him or her to find models outside the session to emulate. Keeping these definitions in mind, pick any two scenarios from this chapter and show how you might apply inadvertent modeling. Then, either using the same scenarios or two different scenarios, demonstrate intentional modeling.

XIV. Confrontation: Support and Challenge

It has been generally assumed that clients should only be confronted when there is a strong base of support already formed. In addition, one's confrontational style can run from moralistic preaching to advance empathy, where you reflect back aspects of the client's experience of which he or she is not aware. For each of the scenarios that follow, develop at least two different ways you might confront the client if you were working with him or her. Consider the following questions when making your responses:

1. Can I confront this person by using advanced empathy?
2. Should I be straightforward with my confrontation?
3. Should I be "heavy handed" in my confrontation?
4. Can I confront this client by pointing out inconsistencies in feelings, actions, and verbalizations?
5. What might be the consequences of a confrontation?
6. Do I need to confront this client at all? Are there alternatives?

Scenarios

1. *Scenario I:* A client, who is making $75,000 a year, tells you that she is in an abusive relationship and cannot move out because she does not have enough money.
2. *Scenario II:* You smell alcohol on the breath of a client who is coming to see you for substance abuse counseling.
3. *Scenario III:* A client whom you have been seeing for a number of months continually tells you that he will work on the counseling "homework" but consistently comes in having done nothing.
4. *Scenario IV:* A client with whom you are working is continually judgmental and critical of others.
5. *Scenario V:* Despite having worked for months with a client, you believe she is not revealing important information that could significantly change the course of counseling.
6. *Scenario VI:* You suspect that your client is having an affair, despite the fact that she tells you she has a "good" marriage.

XV. Often Used Skills (encouragement, affirmations, offering alternatives, information giving, advice giving, collaboration, interpretation, and respectful curiosity)

Below are listed a number of skills that are sometimes used in the counseling relationship. For each skill, write one or two statements describing the skill. Then, using any one scenario from Exercise VII, show how you would make a response using the skill.

1. Encouragement:
    Statement 1_____
    Statement 2_____
    Example_____
_____

2. Affirmations:
    Statement 1_____
    Statement 2_____
    Example_____
_____

3. Offering Alternatives:
    Statement 1_____
    Statement 2_____
    Example_____
_____

4. Information Giving:
    Statement 1_____
    Statement 2_____
    Example_____
_____

5. Advice Giving:
    Statement 1_____
    Statement 2_____
    Example_____
_____

6. Collaboration:
    Statement 1_____
    Statement 2_____
    Example_____
_____

7. Interpretation:
    Statement 1_____
    Statement 2_____
    Example_____
_____

8. Respectful Curiosity
    Statement 1_____
    Statement 2_____
    Example_____
_____

XVI. Assessing Counselor Skills
A. Identifying Often Used Skills with a Client

The following is an interview between a client and counselor. Go through the interview and identify the type of response being made by the helper (empathy, advanced empathy, advice giving, information giving, offering alternatives, confrontation, self-disclosure, modeling, open questions, closed questions, encouragement, affirmations collaboration, referral, and/or summarizing). Each response may have more than one answer. Check the end of this section for the answers.

1. Client: I woke up this morning feeling depressed. My life is out of sorts, and I'm not sure why. Do you think this is something that will pass?

1. Counselor: So, it seems as if your depression just came out of nowhere, and you're not sure what's causing it.

2. Client: Well, yeah. I guess I haven't been real happy lately. I've been in the same relationship now for 15 years, and I just feel like it's dead.

2. Counselor: So it's your relationship that seems to be bringing about most of your sad feelings.

3. Client: That's true. You know, maybe I need to focus on what's going on there. What do you think?

3. Counselor: Well, it certainly seems like you are having strong feelings about your relationship and that you're wondering about whether or not to spend some energy on it.

4. Client: Yeah, I guess in the back of my mind I've known that things have not been going well. Maybe I need to talk to my partner, or suggest relationship counseling, or maybe even just leave!

4. Counselor: What do you think about all those ideas you have?

5. Client: Well, I guess in the back of my mind I've thought about all of those options. But maybe the best place to start would be to have a heart-to-heart talk with my partner. That would be at least a beginning.

5. Counselor: Overall, do you think you feel positive or negative about your relationship?

6. Client: Well, I don't know if it's either. Perhaps more neutral. Sometimes it feels like it doesn't even exist, and other times I feel really close.

6. Counselor: So sometimes you kind of don't feel anything about the relationship while other times you feel like there's a real closeness.

7. Client: That kind of describes it. Maybe I do really need to talk with my partner and see where things are at with both of us.

7. Counselor: How do you think that would be for you?

8. Client: Well, I think it would be difficult, but overall I believe it would be best for us. I mean, I know I have lots of mixed feelings and I would guess my partner does also. In either case, an airing of the situation makes sense.

8. Counselor: Well, it seems that you feel this is the best route for you.

9. Client: Yeah, I guess I do. Although, you know, I'll get pretty nervous opening this whole thing up. But I do think it's best.

9. Counselor: Although I know it might be difficult, I'm encouraged by your desire to work this thing through, one way or another. I know you can make this happen!

10. Client: Yes! I can do it. But you know, I've never been that good at really being straight with people. I think that's because my parents were never real with me, and unfortunately, that's who I've become—I'm not real with others.

10. Counselor: So, you see this as a pattern in your life; that is, that your parents modeled a way of being and that you have taken this same way on in many of your relationships, a way that you do not consider to be particularly good for you.

11. Client: I never really thought it through like this before. But, yeah, I think it goes back to my parents. They always seemed so elusive; I wish I knew them in deeper ways. Now that their dead, I'll never really know who they are (sobbing).

11. Counselor: Well, you're bringing up some really important issues for yourself; some hurts from your childhood that seem to affect your relationships today.

12. Client: Maybe I'm really much sicker than I thought. What do you think?

12. Counselor: I think you're struggling with some important issues in your life. Some very painful ones.

13. Client: Yes, I guess so.

13. Counselor: I admire your wanting to work on these issues.

14. Client: I guess I really need to examine some of this stuff. I tend to blame my partner for some of my issues, and maybe it's related more to some stuff of my own—not that she doesn't have some issues also.

14. Counselor: You know, I had some problems once in my life that were really difficult for me. Working on them made me feel better about who I am and gave me more insight into my relationships.

15. Client: Really?

15. Counselor: Yeah, it was really helpful for me. I know you can move on in your life in a positive way and feel good about you. You have all the ingredients in you to make this work.

16. Client: I hope so. I think this is a really good start. Can I talk about one other thing?

16. Counselor: Sure.

17. Client: I notice that on some nights, not all nights mind you, I seem to drink a lot. I wake up in the morning feeling terrible. I wonder if this affects my work performance. I've been thinking about maybe trying out an AA meeting. What do you think?

17. Counselor: I hear your concern about your drinking and the fact that you have been giving some serious thought to doing something about it.

18. Client: To be honest, sometimes I really think I go overboard with my drinking.

18. Counselor: Well, it sounds to me as if you might have a problem with alcohol and perhaps you should do something about it.

19. Client: Do you know of any AA meetings?

19. Counselor: Yep, let me give you a list I have right here. You know, AA meetings usually last a couple of hours and one's anonymity is ensured. I have heard that people who go to AA meetings are usually accepting of one another.

20. Client: Well, you've been helpful. I appreciate all of what you've done for me.

20. Counselor: Thanks. I hear that you are ready to do some important things for you. For instance, today you talked about some concerns you have with your relationship with your partner. You also noted that perhaps some of these are related to some issues you had with your parents growing up. You thought that perhaps their inability to be real with you affected how you are in relationships. Finally, you talked about a possible problem with drinking and we located some AA meetings you could go to. I'd like to hear your thoughts about what we did today and about setting some goals. Maybe together, we can agree on the direction we want this to go.

21. Client: That sounds good. I have some thoughts about what I should do, and I certainly want to hear your thoughts.

21. Counselor: All in all, you did a lot of work today. Good for you!

Answers to Exercise XVI.A: (1) empathy, (2) empathy, (3) empathy, (4) open question, (5) closed question, (6) empathy, (7) open question, (8) empathy, (9) encouragement, (10) advanced empathy, (11) advanced empathy, (12) empathy, (13) affirmation, (14) self-disclosure, modeling , (15) self-esteem building, (16) not ratable, (17) empathy, (18) mild confrontation, (19) referrals, information giving, (20) summarizing, collaboration, (21) affirmation.

B. Identifying Solution-Focused Brief Skills

Exercise XVI.A used a number of traditional skills in working with the client. This exercise uses solution-focused brief skills in working with the same client. As you go through the abridged interview, pick out the following skills often used in solution-focused brief therapy: empathy, respectful curiosity, coping questions, exception-seeking questions, the miracle question, and collaboration. Check the end of this section for the answers.

1. Client: I woke up this morning feeling depressed. My life is out of sorts, and I'm not sure why. Do you think this is something that will pass?
1. Counselor: I am hopeful that this is something you can overcome. Let's see if we can work together to find some solutions to your problems. I wonder if you can tell me a little more about the depression.
2. Client: Well, I guess I haven't been real happy lately. I've been in the same relationship now for 15 years, and I just feel like it's dead.
2. Counselor: That must feel horrible. Is it that you're thinking the relationship is a major source of your depression?
3. Client: Yes, you know, maybe I need to focus in on what's going on there. What do you think?
3. Counselor: Well, I guess I'm wondering when you felt like you handled your depression well—times when you seemed to be able to overcome those sad feelings.
4. Client: It seems like the times I felt best were when my wife and I were talking more and when I was feeling much healthier, physically.
4. Counselor: Can you tell me about those times? What was it like when you and your wife talked more and you felt better physically?
5. Client: I wasn't drinking as much, for one. I think the drinking has become a real solace for me. You know, I drink to rid myself of my sad feelings. Or maybe, I feel sad because I drink. I don't know.
5. Counselor: In either case, you coped well when you were feeling healthier and drinking less. Is that about right?
6. Client: Yes. Definitely.
6. Counselor: And what else enabled you to feel better in those times?
7. Client: Well, we had children living with us then, and I think we both focused in on them a lot, rather than on just the relationship.
7. Counselor: So if I'm hearing you right, not drinking, focusing on the children, and generally feeling healthier all made it an easier time for you. Can you also think about times when you did not have this problem? What was that like?
8. Client: Interesting question. You know, before I retired, my problems seemed much less important. I had other things to worry about—well, not even worry, but to spend time on. You know, like my work, my kids, and even my wife. I mean, going out on a "date" was an event then.

8. Counselor: Well, you talked about a bunch of things that seemed to make you feel better or ways that you were able to cope better in the past. Let me ask you something, if you were to wake up tomorrow morning and your life were "fixed" and you no longer felt depressed, what would your life look like?

9. Client: Another interesting question! Let me think. I believe that if things were fixed, I would not be drinking, I would have a hobby, and maybe even I would take wife out on a date once in a while.

9. Counselor: Interesting. Any ideas how you might be able to make that happen?

10. Client: Well, yeah. My buddy goes to AA meetings, and I can certainly join him. And, I've been thinking about getting involved in a model airplane club. And, you know, I really do need to tend to my wife a bit more.

10. Counselor: Well, it sounds like you've come up with some good solutions, rather quickly. Why don't you start on some of those ideas, and we can meet again in a bit and see how it's going? Does that sound good to you?

11. Client: Sounds really good. Thanks….

Answers to Exercise XVI.B: (1) respectful curiosity, collaboration, (2) empathy, respectful curiosity (3) coping question, (4) respectful curiosity, (5) respectful curiosity, empathy (6) coping question (7) empathy, exception-seeking question (8) empathy, miracle question (9) respectful curiosity (10) collaboration.

C. Comparing Often Used Skills and Solution-Focused Skills

These days, counselors are often encouraged to use skills that are brief, such as the solution-focused skills in Exercise B. In small groups, compare and contrast the more traditional skills in Exercise B with those skills in Exercise C. What might be the advantages and disadvantages of both? Which are you more comfortable using?

XVII. The Good vs. the Bad Counselor

Have students break into triads, and have one student be number 1, a second student be number 2, and a third student be number 3. Ask number 1 to play a bad counselor, and have that individual give any response he or she so chooses (e.g., advice giving, closed questions, being critical, being overly confrontational). Number 2 should role-play the client. After that role-play is complete, have number 2 role-play a good counselor and number 3 play a client. The person who is not given a role can be an observer, offering feedback at the end of the mini-session. Do these role-plays for 5 or 10 minutes at a time, and if time allows, switch roles (i.e., have number 3 play the bad counselor and number 1 the good counselor, etc.). At the end of the exercise, students should share their responses in class and compare and contrast the effectiveness of good vs. bad counselor responses.

* This exercise was adapted from material by Dr. Paula Bickham, who is in private practice in Charleston, WV and developing a post-masters training program.. Her contribution is greatly appreciated.

XVIII. Writing Case Notes
A. Basic Case Notes

Using the interview in Exercise XVIA and/or XVIB, write case notes of your contact with this client and make recommendations for future sessions. Keep your case notes to one page and make sure they are objective, nonjudgmental, focused on the major issues, and offer direction for future sessions.

B. SOAP Notes

These days, many counseling settings encourage counselors to use SOAP notes, which offer a systematic way of gathering information and organizing the information you obtained from your client during a session. Using Table 5.1, role-play with a student in class, and when you are finished, using this format, write your case notes in the "comments" section Table 5.1.

IXX. Writing Case Reports

Meet with another student and role-play two problem situations, with one student being the counselor the first time and the other student being the counselor during the second role-play. Then, based on your role-play, and using some or all of the categories often addressed in a clinical case report as found in Appendix E, write a two- to four-page report. Your instructor will highlight those categories in Appendix E that he or she feels are important for you at this point in your course work.

XX. Ethical, Legal, and Professional Vignettes

(The ACA's code is at www.counseling.org under "Resources"). In responding to the following, consider referring to the ACA's code.

For the following vignettes, write some possible solutions and be prepared to discuss them in class.

A. Case Note Security

1. A client who is coming to your agency demands to see her case notes. In them, you have noted that you suspect she may be lying about her Social Security eligibility and that you also suspect she might be paranoid. What do you do?
2. A client you have been seeing at a crisis center comes in and asks to see all records pertaining to him. These include crisis logs that have information in them about other clients, as well as case notes you have made concerning his contacts. Does this client have a right to his records? What should you do?
3. You suspect that a colleague of yours is sharing information about his clients with close friends. Since this is unethical, how should you handle the situation?

B. Confidentiality and Primary Obligation: Client, Agency, or Society

4. You're working at an agency that specializes in outpatient counseling for substance abuse. In the course of a conversation with a client, you discover that she has been using crystal meth. An agency dictate states that any client suspected of using illegal drugs must be immediately referred to rehabilitation, and if he or she refuses, you can no longer see the client at your agency. You explain this to her, she gets angry, walks out, and states she'll "blow this place up." What do you do?
5. In your conversation with a client at the day treatment center where you work, you discover that he is drinking and taking large amounts of a tranquilizer, and you suspect he may be considering killing himself. You ask him about this, and he tells you to mind your own business. What do you do?

Table 5.1: SOAP Case Notes

S	Subjective-Description	Subjective-Examples	Subjective-Pointers
	• What the client tells you (feelings, concerns, plans, goals, thoughts) • How the client experiences the world • Client's orientation to time, place, and person	• Client reports… • Client shares…. • Client describes… • Client indicates…	• Avoid quotations • Full names of others are generally not needed • Be concise • Limit adjectives
Comments:			

O	Objective-Description	Objective-Examples	Objective-Pointers
	• Factual: what the helper personally observes and/or witnesses • Quantifiable: what was seen, heard, smelled, counted, or measured (may include outside written materials)	• Appeared _____ as evidenced by…. • Test results indicate… • Client's hair uncombed; clothes unkempt	• Avoid words like client "appeared" or "seemed" when not supported by objective examples • Avoid labels, personal judgments, or opinionated statements
Comments:			

A	Assessment-Description	Assessment-Examples	Assessment-Pointers
	• Summarizes the helper's clinical thinking • Includes diagnoses or clinical impressions and reasons for behavior	• Behavior/attitude consistent with individuals who…. • DSM-IV-TR diagnosis • Rule out…	• May note themes, or recurring issues • Remain professional • Remember that others may view assessment
Comments:			

P	Plan-Description	Plan-Examples	Plan-Pointers
	• Describes parameters of treatment • Includes action plan; interventions; progress; prognosis; treatment direction for next session.	• Counselor established rapport, challenged, etc. • Client progress is indicated by… • Next session, counselor will… • Client and counselor will continue to…	• Give supporting reasons for progress • "Progress is fair due to client's inconsistent attendance at sessions"
Comments:			

Adapted from: Cameron, S., & turtle-song, i. (2002). Learning to write case notes using the SOAP format. *Journal of Counseling & Development, 80*(3), 286-92.

6. In the course of working with a client, she expresses her concern about her grandmother who, she states, lives by herself, is depressed, has stopped eating, and has lost a considerable amount of weight. You contact her, but she refuses services. What do you do?
7. While talking with a 15-year-old male client, he informs you that on a recent vacation he was sexually molested by an uncle. He asks you not to tell his parents. What do you do?
8. A 15-year-old client tells you he is having sexual relations with his 14-year-old stepsister. What do you do?
9. An adult client informs you that he wants to kill his ex-girlfriend and her new boyfriend. He denies that he actually will act on these feelings but that he just "thinks about it a lot." What do you do?

C. Competence
10. A colleague of yours tells you that she is going to try out a new psychotherapeutic technique that involves untested therapeutic strategies. She has not been trained in the procedures, but a recent best-selling book speaks to the success of it. Do you have any obligation to prevent her from trying this new approach?
11. A colleague of yours has decided to refer to you the son of a family he has been seeing in family therapy. With permission from the parents, he sends to you his case notes on the family sessions for background information. You read the case notes and believe that he has been acting incompetently during the session. What should you do?

D. Fees
12. A client is referred to a private practitioner for individual counseling. After discovering that the client does not have insurance that covers mental health concerns and that the client cannot afford to pay, the counselor refers the client to the local community mental health center. Has the counselor acted ethically? Is this professional? Is this legal?
13. The parents of a school counselor decide to give the counselor a $50 gift certificate to a local restaurant for the work she has done with their child. Should the counselor accept the gift?
14. A college counselor who has been consulting with a faculty member concerning some problem students is given a relatively expensive gift by the faculty member. Should the counselor accept this gift? Is this ethical? Professional?
15. A client complains to her licensed professional counselor that she did not know she would have to pay for sessions that were not covered by her insurance company. Under what circumstances, if any, does the counselor have the right to sue the client for lack of payment?
16. A counselor decides to ask a collection agency to try and recover money from past and current clients who have an outstanding balance. Is this ethical? Professional? Legal?

E. Multiple Relationships
17. A client you have been working with for a number of months invites you to her wedding. You are both concerned about the multiple relationships involved with going to the wedding, but also believe that if you go, there is potential to build a

stronger relationship with your client. What is your ethical obligation? What should you do?

18. A client's father dies; you have been working with her for a number of months, and you know that it would mean much to her if you went to the funeral. Should you go? What is your ethical obligation? How might this issue be different from the one in Item 17?

F. End-of-Life Counseling

19. Your client is in the final stages of cancer and death is imminent. She is in considerable pain, and tells you that she is considering ending her life with the vial of morphine given to her by hospice. The vial is for pain reduction, but if she takes it all, she will die. What should you do? What is your ethical obligation? What is your legal responsibility?

CHAPTER 6

COUPLES AND FAMILY COUNSELING

I. General Systems Theory

General systems theory (Bertalanfy, 1968) was developed to explain the complex interactions of all types of systems, including living systems, family systems, community systems, and solar systems. With this in mind, discuss the following:

1. What similar systemic properties can you find among the ecosystem, family system, social system, and solar system?
2. All systems are said to have boundaries. What might be some of the properties of a system that has rigid boundaries (i.e., does not allow information to flow in or out)? Loosely structured or diffuse boundaries? Semi-permeable boundaries?
3. Describe what might occur in any system if a major component is somehow disrupted or made to act differently. Then, reflect on the ways in which a disruption might affect a family.
4. In class, discuss or role-play a family that has rigid boundaries, loose or diffuse boundaries, and semi-permeable boundaries.
5. Using some of the rules of general systems theory, discuss some of the characteristics of a healthy family and contrast those with characteristics of a dysfunctional family.
6. In dyads, identify someone with whom you have had a significant conflict. Now, discuss with the other person your contribution to the conflict. Remember, your contribution may have occurred earlier in the relationship or may involve an unconscious issue with that person. Are you able to see how the conflict is circular and reciprocal?[1]

II. Cybernetics

The study of *cybernetics*, or control mechanisms in systems, has been used to explain the regulatory process of a system and is closely related to the systems' *homeostasis*. One type of cybernetic system is the thermostat. As it becomes colder, the temperature drops, and the thermostat turns on the heating system; as the temperature goes up, the thermostat shuts down the heat. This type of cybernetic system is called a *negative feedback loop* because it keeps the irregularities within the system at a minimum. *Positive feedback loops* are when change in one component in a system leads to a change in another component within the same system, which leads to a change in the first component, and so on. On the relationship level, cybernetics explains how couples and families regulate themselves using their unique ways of communicating as they maintain their homeostasis. With this in mind, have two people role-play a couple that has a negative feedback loop kick in when they argue. Then, have two people role-play a couple that has a positive feedback loop kick in when they argue. Discuss the differences. Which couple do you think would be easier to work with?

---

[1] Exercise 6 was adapted from an exercise by Dr. Jered Kolbert, from Slippery Rock University. His contribution is greatly appreciated.

III. Applying an Understanding of Systems to Your Family

Box 6.1 provides 12 statements that often are applied to an understanding of couples and family counseling. For each statement, see if you can describe how the statement applies to your family of origin. Share your answers in small groups in class.

Box 6.1: Understanding Couples and Family Counseling

1. The interactional forces between couples and in families are complex, and cannot be explained in a simple, causal fashion.
2. Couples and families have overt and covert rules that govern their functioning.
3. Understanding the complementary nature of couples and the hierarchy in a family (e.g., who's "in charge"; who makes the rules) can help one understand the makeup and communication sequences of couples and of families.
4. Comprehension of the boundaries and subsystems (e.g., spousal, sibling) of couples or families can help one understand the makeup and communication sequences of a couple and of a family.
5. Understanding whether boundaries are rigid, diffuse, or semi-permeable (e.g., how information can get in and out of couples and families) can help one make sense of how communication and change occur in couples and in families.
6. Understanding how couples and family members communicate can give insight into how couples and families maintain their way of functioning.
7. Each couple and family has its own unique homeostasis that describes how its members typically interact. This homeostasis is not "bad" or "good." It simply is.
8. Communication in couples and families is complex, and the language they use tells a message about who they are.
9. Change occurs by changing the homeostasis, or the usual patterns, in the couple and in the family.
10. Issues passed down by language in families, in culture, and in society affect how couples and families come to define themselves.
11. Stress from the expected developmental milestones (marriage, birth of a child, etc.) can wreak havoc on a couple and family, so counselors should be aware of the particular issues involved in such developmental crises.
12. In addition to being equipped to deal with stress from developmental milestones, couples and family counselors should have the tools to help couples and families deal with the unexpected stressors of life.

IV. The Power of Language in Family Development

In recent years, much notice has been placed on the power of language in the development of families. Some suggest that those who are in positions of power (the "majority") subtly, and sometimes not so subtly, develop a language system along with laws and policies that support this system, to forward their agenda. This agenda usually is oppressive of disenfranchised or nondominant groups and results in more power and wealth for the majority. With this in mind, in ethnically/culturally diverse small groups, discuss the following questions:

1. How might language in American culture oppress certain groups?
2. Can you identify any policies or laws that have specifically been detrimental to the development of families from nondominant groups?
3. What language do you use that may subtly oppress others?

4. Do you believe that even nondominant groups may sometimes "buy into" the very oppressive language of dominant groups (e.g., an anti-gay individual who has bought into anti-gay rhetoric, suddenly realizes he's gay)?

V. Situational Stress in Families
A. Types of Situational Stress
In the life of all families, unique situations will arise with which families must cope (death of a sibling, illness, divorce). Make a list of some kinds of issues that could arise in the development of a family, including any situational issues that your family of origin may have experienced. Share your lists in class.

B. Reactions to Situational Stress
In small groups, discuss differences in the ways a healthy family might deal with situational stress as compared to a dysfunctional family. If you feel comfortable, discuss how your family of origin dealt with situational issues that affected it.

VI. Reflecting on Your Family of Origin
Reflect on your family of origin, and write responses to the following questions:
1. What roles did members of your family take on as you were growing up?
2. Do you think your family had rigid, loose (diffuse), or semi-permeable boundaries?
3. Were there predictable patterns of behavior that you could identify in the various members of your family?
4. What would happen if a member of your family acted differently than expected?
5. Was there a family member who was scapegoated and/or an identified patient?
6. How did your family handle conflict?
7. When your family experienced periods of stress, how was it handled?
8. What situational stress did you or members of your family experience? How was it handled?
9. What developmental cycles do you recall, and how did your family handle them?
10. How might the language (nonverbal and verbal) used in your family affect how each family member came to understand his or her place in the world?

VII. Family Development
A. Developmental Stages of Family
All families pass through normal and predictable developmental stages. For instance, Table 6.1 shows a list of the developmental stages families typically pass through. For each developmental stage, list some difficulties typically faced by families and then describe how they might need to adjust to the changes as a result of developmental shifts (see examples in the first two stages). Share what you wrote in small groups and/or in class.

B. Other Developmental Theories
Choose any developmental theory (e.g., Erikson, 1963, 1980, 1982; Gilligan, 1982; Kohlberg, 1969, 1984), and discuss how specific developmental stages may affect the development of the family and extended family.

C. Your Family of Origin
Using Table 6.1 or one of the developmental theories in "B," discuss how your family of origin dealt with predictable developmental stages.

Table 6.1: Family Developmental Stages

Stage	Typical Problems Faced by Families	How People/Families Adjust
Partnering (e.g., Marriage)	1. Negotiating living space with new person 2. Dealing with differences in values 3. 4.	1. Argue/fight 2. Find new ways of communicating and compromising 3. 4.
Having Children	1. Learning how to nurture 2. Learning how to discipline 3. 4.	1. Arguing/discussing ways of parenting 2. 3. 4.
Children Entering Elementary School	1. 2. 3. 4.	1. 2. 3. 4.
Children Entering Adolescence	1. 2. 3. 4.	1. 2. 3. 4.
Children, Now Young Adults, Leaving Home	1. 2. 3. 4.	1. 2. 3. 4.
Adults Moving into Mid and Later Life	1. 2. 3. 4.	1. 2. 3. 4.
Aging Parent(s)	1. 2. 3. 4.	1. 2. 3. 4.

VIII. Your Family Genogram
A. Creating Your Genogram
Using the genogram in Figure 6.1 as a model, create your own family genogram that goes back at least two generations. Consider including additional information other than what is on this genogram, such as place of birth, cause of death, genetic illnesses, mental retardation, mental illness, and so forth.

B. Sharing Your Genogram
After having completed your genogram, sit down with another student in class and discuss your family of origin. Pay particular notice to any patterns of behavior, or significant events that may have affected the ways in which your family interacted. After both of you have shared your genograms with one another, highlight a couple of important facts that each of you learned about the other and share those in class.

C. Cross-Cultural Differences
After you have learned about other students' genograms, do you notice any cross-cultural patterns? For instance, is there a tendency for students from some ethnic/cultural groups to be first-generation college students? Are some cultural groups' extended family more important to the family decision-making process than others? And so forth. Discuss in class.

IX. Working with a Family in Need
Box 6.2 describes a family that sought aid from an agency. Read about the family, and then respond to the following questions:
1. Do you think this family's boundaries are rigid, loose, or semi-permeable?
2. Do you believe that any member(s) of this family is (are) being scapegoated?
3. Is there an identified patient (IP) in this family?
4. What counseling skills would you need to have to work effectively with this family?
5. How would you diagnose the problem areas in this family?
6. What needs does this family have?
7. What goals would you help the family set for itself?
8. What referrals would be appropriate for this family?
9. What type of follow-up would you want to do?
10. What societal pressures do you think have negatively affected this family?
11. Do you have any obligation to contact Child Protective Services for this family?

X. Comparing and Contrasting Family Therapy Approaches
In class, your instructor will have small groups assigned to some or all of the family therapy approaches listed below. In your small groups, discuss how you would work with the family in Box 6.2. Share what you discuss with the class.
1. Human validation process model (Satir)
2. Structural family therapy (Minuchin)
3. Strategic family therapy (Haley, Madanes)
4. Multigenerational approaches (Bowen; Boszormenyi-Nagy)
5. Experiential family therapy (Whitaker, Napier)
6. Psychodynamic family therapy (Ackerman)
7. Behavioral and cognitive-behavioral family therapy
8. Narrative family therapy (White, Epston)
9. Solution-focused family therapy (de Shazer, Berg, O'Hanlon)

Figure 6.1: Williams-Neukrug Genogram

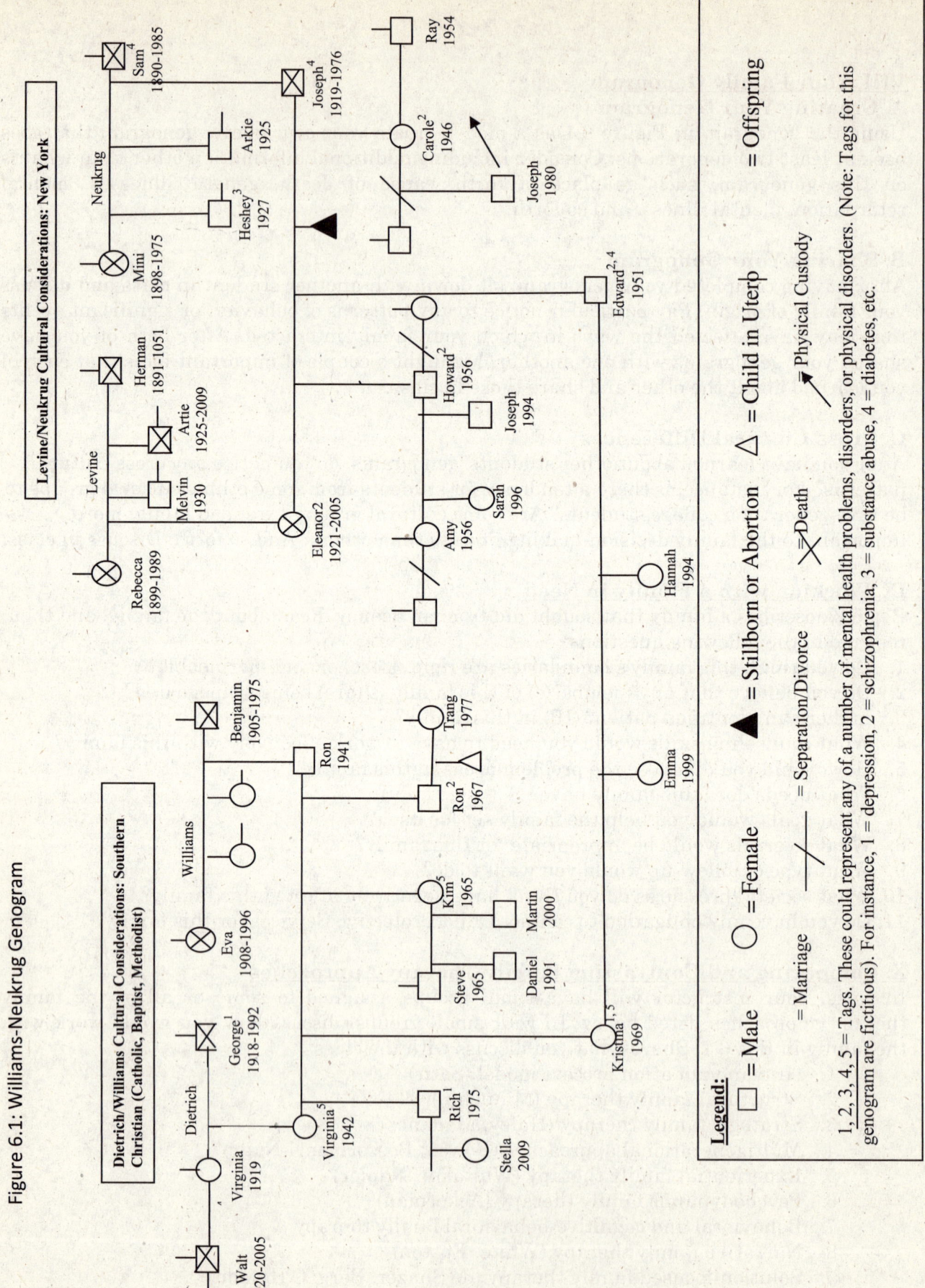

> **BOX 6.2: David, Jan, and Children**
>
> David, Jan, and their three children have just moved to the area. They made the move because David thought he would have an easier time finding a job. Having left family and friends, they no longer have the support that they had at their prior residence. They noted that when they first moved, they were living out of their car and then at the "hotel from hell," but they recently moved into a low-income subsidized housing project. David is an unemployed construction worker, and Jan works part time at the local convenience store. David is 28 and Jan is 29. They have been married 10 years. Jan states that David "sometimes drinks too much"; David denies this. David states that Jan has "gotten too fat"; Jan admits having gained some weight but states that "David should love me anyway." During your meeting with them, you find that they often argue with each other about work, the children, and Jan's weight.
>
> Mark, the oldest child, is 11 and has been autistic from birth. Jan and David have received disability for him in the past and previously placed him in a residential treatment center. They are unsure about how to care for him now that they have moved. Jordan, who is 9 years old, has had behavioral problems in school and has been involved in some vandalism in his neighborhood. Jan thinks he may be "drug running" for some of the older kids in the neighborhood. Jordan is entering the third grade (he was held back a year at his previous school). David and Jan are unclear on how to register Jordan in his new school. In fact, they're not sure where his new school is located. They describe their youngest child, Jessica, as "their gem." She is 6 years old and entering the first grade. They state that she is the only one who has not caused them problems.
>
> Jan and David attempt to control their children through punishment, and you suspect child abuse may be occurring in the family. You also suspect that there may be secrets in the family as the children seem scared to openly talk during a session. When you meet with the family, David attempts to control everyone by demanding compliance and by yelling. Jan will periodically shake a child if he or she is misbehaving during a session.

XI. Role-Playing Family Therapy

Your instructor will ask one or more students to volunteer to present a family problem that occurred in their family of origin. Then, pairs of students will be asked to be co-therapists as other members of the class role-play one or more of the families discussed in class. Co-therapists should use one of the theoretical orientations listed in Exercise IX and/or a family therapy approach discussed in class.

XII. Comparing Individual and Family Therapy Approaches

Box 6.3 describes Alice, an individual who has sought aid from your agency. Read the description, and then respond to the following questions:
1. Do you believe Alice should be counseled individually or in family counseling? Why?
2. From a systemic perspective, how might you describe Alice's problems?

3. If you were viewing Alice's situation from an individualistic perspective, would your understanding of Alice's predicament change?
4. What risks are involved in working with Alice from a family perspective?
5. What risks are involved in working with Alice from an individualistic perspective?
6. How might you proceed with Alice if you were to work with her in family counseling?
7. What counseling skills would you need to work effectively with Alice if you were to work with her in family counseling?
8. What goals would you help Alice set for herself?

Box 6.3: Alice

Alice is a 16-year-old single female who is three months pregnant. She seeks your advice concerning her pregnancy. She lives with her parents and her 15-year-old sister. She has not told her parents about the pregnancy and is concerned that, before long, they will find out. Her family has little money, and she is worried about having enough money to pay the medical expenses for the pregnancy and birth. Her parents do not have medical insurance. Alice has come to you because she feels depressed and at the "end of her rope." She is looking for help. When you meet with her, she sobs throughout the interview and at times seems to whine.

Alice's 36-year-old father Arnold is a part-time truck driver. Alice states that he has rigid views and tends to be rather "authoritarian." She also thinks that he will "lose it" if he learns she is pregnant and will want to "take care of the situation" to make it go away. Although he has not physically abused her in the past two years, when she was younger, he would often "take a belt to me." At times, he drinks too much, and there seem to be conflicts between him and his wife. He was married at age 18.

Alice states that her mother "cares a lot about me"; however, she also notes that her mother would never go against her father's wishes. Alice's mother Linda, who is 35 years old, works part time at a fast food restaurant and is very concerned about her daughter's well-being. Because she got married when she was pregnant with Alice, Alice thinks that her mother will probably understand her situation.

Joan is Alice's 15-year-old sister. Alice states that Joan is a good student but at time acts like a "wise-ass." She feels as if Joan has always received all the attention in the family; now that she is pregnant, Alice is concerned that she will be even more of an outcast. Alice notes that Joan has many friends and is often out of the house doing things rather than staying home with her "drunk dad" and her mom.

XIII. Professional Associations
1. Compare and contrast the International Association of Marriage and Family Therapy (IAMFC; http://www.iamfconline.com/), which is a division of the ACA, with the Association of Marriage and Family Therapy (AAMFT; http://www.amft.org).
2. Find the codes of ethics of both professional associations and compare them. How are they similar or different?
3. If you were to join just one of the associations, which would you pick? Why?

IV. Ethical, Legal, and Professional Vignettes

(The ACA's code is at www.counseling.org under "Resources"). In responding to the following, consider referring to the ACA's code.

1. A counselor is contacted by Mrs. Jay, who is concerned about the behavior of her 12-year-old son. She states that he is "acting odd, seems like he doesn't care about anything, and doesn't listen to anyone about anything." She also believes that he has been lying to her about "all different kinds of things." The counselor states to Mrs. Jay that he would be glad to meet with the whole family and discuss the problem, at which point Mrs. Jay states that she could never get her husband to come in for counseling. She goes on to state that her 10-year-old daughter could come, but "isn't the problem with Jamille." The counselor states that when one member in the family has a problem, all of the family has a problem and goes on to assert that he will not see the son without the whole family being present. Mrs. Jay says she'll see what she can do. At the time of the first session, Mrs. Jay shows up with her son and daughter but states that her husband would not come in. The counselor insists on seeing the whole family, does not interview Mrs. Jay and the children, and sets up another appointment time. No one shows up for the next appointment. Despite further attempts to get the family in, the counselor is not successful. Has the counselor acted ethically? Professionally?

2. Prior to seeing a family for counseling, a counselor gives a written document explaining the process of counseling to the parents. After reading this *informed consent* document, the parents sign it and bring the family to counseling. The informed consent document is not given to or described to the children. Has the counselor acted ethically? Professionally?

3. A wife/mother who is seeing you in family counseling calls and starts to describe how depressed she is. During your next family session, you reveal to the family that the wife/mother is extremely depressed. Is this breaking of confidentiality ethical? Is it the professional thing to do? Is it legal?

4. Referring to vignette number 3, what if the woman called and told you she was having an affair? Would the breaking of confidentiality in this instance be of a different nature than in vignette 3?

5. You are seeing a family in family counseling when you realize the father is extremely depressed, perhaps suicidally so. You decide to see him for individual sessions and to continue the family sessions. Is this ethical? Is this the professional thing to do?

6. A colleague of yours is seeing a family for family counseling. The health insurance company to which the family belongs allows each member of the family to have 10 sessions for individual counseling and does not provide payments for family therapy. You therefore decide to sequentially bill each member of the family so you can continue to see them in family counseling. Is this ethical? Is this professional? Is this legal?

7. After meeting for a few sessions with a middle school student, a school counselor determines that the student is severely disturbed due to a dysfunctional family system. The counselor would prefer to see the whole family, but the school system frowns upon family counseling. The counselor therefore decides to continue to work individually with the student. Is this ethical? Is this the professional thing to do?

8. Suppose that the school counselor in vignette 7 had referred the family to a local community agency for family counseling. Under what circumstances might it be ethical for the counselor to continue to see the student for individual sessions while the student was also being seen for family therapy at the community agency?

9. In deciding how to act on an ethical concern, a counselor notices that the code of ethics of the American Association for Marriage and Family Therapy (AAMFT) has a different response to a situation than the code of ethics of the International Association of Marriage and Family Counselors (IAMFC). The counselor decides to go with the code of ethics that best matches her view of the situation. Is this ethical? Is this the professional thing to do?
10. After working with a couple for six months in marital counseling, they decide to separate. A few months later, the counselor is subpoenaed to testify against one of the spouses. Does the counselor have to testify?
11. A counselor you know is practicing family counseling, even though you believe she has major issues that are unfinished from her family of origin. Is this ethical? Is this professional? What obligation do you have, if any, in this situation?
12. A couple seeks out counseling for their adolescent child whose grades have significantly dropped in school. They also tell you that they believe their child is depressed. You begin to see the whole family, which consists of a grandmother, the couple, and three children. After the second session, the mother calls and wants to discuss the progress of the child that brought them to counseling. The counselor states that the problem goes further than the child and that she would prefer to discuss it in front of the whole family. Has the counselor acted ethically? Has the counselor acted in a professional manner?
13. A counselor who has graduated from a school accredited by the American Association of Marriage and Family Therapists decides to open a practice as a marriage and family counselor, despite the fact that he is not licensed in his state. Is this ethical? Is this professional? Is this legal?
14. A counselor becomes certified as a family counselor through the National Academy for Certified Family Therapists. She advertises herself as a certified family therapist and opens a practice. She is not licensed by her state. Is this ethical? Is this professional? Is this legal?

CHAPTER 7

GROUP WORK

I. Groups as a System

Using the attributes below, compare your family of origin with a group in which you have participated. When you are finished, discuss whether you believe groups and families are similar to one another in the ways they function.

a. Cohesiveness
b. Information flow
c. Boundaries
d. Organization (e.g., subgroups, hierarchies)
e. Scapegoating and/or identified patients
f. Ability to change

II. Wearing Labels

Your instructor will cut out each of the phrases listed below (or others of his or her choice) and without telling which one, tape one on each student's forehead. After your instructor is finished, find an open space and mill around, responding to others based on the phrase they have on their foreheads. After a few minutes, sit in a large circle, and without removing the phrase, discuss how people interacted with you. Try to identify the label you were wearing.

Look at me intensely.
Tell me you like what I'm wearing.
Frown at me. Act as if I don't exist.
Yell at me when I speak.
Be angry at me.
Treat me humanely.
Act disgusted toward me.
Talk to me but don't listen to me.
Treat me like an object when you talk to me.
Act as if you like me even though you don't.

Walk away from me.
Look at my shoes.
Be loving toward me.
Speak softly to me.
Look at my stomach.
Touch me when you talk to me.
Be nice to me. Be rude to me.
Disagree with anything I say.
Reflect back anything I say.

After the class has finished the exercise, discuss the following questions:
1. What's it like being labeled?
2. Do we all wear labels as we go through life? (Are there certain personality characteristics that we tend to exhibit?)
3. If we do exhibit certain personality characteristics, is it possible that we create other people's responses to us by these personality characteristics?
4. How can the group process help us understand the labels (personality characteristics) that we exhibit?
5. How easy is it to change our labels, and subsequently, the ways we interact with others?

III. Advantages and Disadvantages of Groups

In the space provided, write in as many advantages and disadvantages as you can of group counseling when compared to individual counseling. Share your responses in class.

Advantages	Disadvantages
_____	_____
_____	_____
_____	_____
_____	_____
_____	_____

IV. Ecological Concepts in Groups

Discuss in small groups:
1. Seating arrangement is one critical factor in helping group members feel safe and build cohesion. Describe what you think is the optimal seating arrangement.
2. What additional environmental factors can affect group cohesion?
3. Describes the kinds of interactions you believe would occur among group members that would increase group trust and productivity?
4. What are some examples of therapeutic conditions that enhance a positive social system and group interconnections?
5. If a group leader facilitates understanding about self and others, one gains an increased sense of meaning (Conyne, Crowell, & Newmeyer, 2008).
    a. What kind of techniques do you think would facilitate this experience?
    b. How does a leader determine if group members are having this experience?

* This exercise was adapted from material by Dr. Jeri Crowell, Capella University and the Southern Center for Choice Theory. Her contribution is greatly appreciated.

V. Comparison of Groups: Free Association

Your instructor will write the five types of groups listed below on the board. Share the first words that come to mind for each of the groups listed. Or, at home, write down the first words that come to mind in the space provided. Discuss your responses in class.

1. Self-help groups _____   4. Counseling groups _____
2. Task groups _____   5. Therapy groups _____
3. Psychoeducational groups _____

VI. Self-Help Groups

A. Sharing Experiences
If you have participated in a self-help group and feel comfortable sharing your experience in class, describe the self-help group with your class.

B. Visiting a Self-Help Group
Visit one open self-help group and share your experience with your classmates (e.g., AA, weight watchers, etc.). Pay particular attention to the following:
1. Is there a person who leads the group? If so, is the leader a trained professional?
2. How often and for what length of time does the group meet?

3. Is there a fee for participation in the group?
4. Describe what takes place in the group.
5. Give your general impressions of the group.

VII. Task Groups
A. Influences on Task Groups
Reflect on any group experience you have had and discuss with others how the group process can be affected by the following attributes of the group members:
1. Age
2. Gender
3. Ethnic/cultural background
4. Expertise and/or educational
5. Disability
6. "Attractiveness"

B. The Shelter
Your instructor will have the class break into groups of six to eight students. Each group will work on the problem in Box 7.1. When you are finished, discuss how the dynamics in your group may have been affected by the factors listed in Exercise A. How were the choices *you* made affected by these same factors?

Box 7.1: The Bomb Shelter

An asteroid has hit Earth, creating an ice-encrusted planet. There are only 10 individuals left on the planet, who survived by going into an old nuclear bomb shelter. It is expected that the planet will, in a few years, return to relative normalcy. However, for the next two years, any attempt to leave the shelter will lead to sure death. There is only enough food and water to last for one year. If four individuals would leave the shelter, there would likely be enough food and water for the other six to survive until the planet was again livable. Your group task is to decide which four individuals out of the following 10 people in the shelter will be asked to leave.

1. A pregnant mentally retarded 15-year-old
2. A Caucasian writer with Parkinson's disease
3. An elderly Orthodox rabbi
4. An alcoholic doctor
5. A physically abusive engineer
6. A gay African-American firefighter
7. A Chinese-American counselor educator
8. An elderly priest who is a steadfast celibate
9. A depressed teacher
10. A farmer who is a member of the Supreme Society for Social Justice (a militia group)

VIII. Developing a Psychoeducational Group (Guidance Group)
Develop an outline of a psychoeducational group on a topic of your choice. Describe the following in the development of your program:
1. The title of the program
2. A brief outline of your program
3. Technical issues related to your program (e.g., open or closed, the frequency of meetings, the length of meetings, the expected duration of the group, meeting place, etc.)
4. Number of participants
5. Ground rules and ethical concerns
6. How you would handle closure of the group
7. Any follow-up you might do

IX. Group Counseling
A. Role-Playing Group Stages
Your instructor will ask 6 to 10 students to role-play a counseling group. In addition, two students will be asked to be co-leaders of the group for a pre-group session, and two will be asked to be co-leaders for each of the stages of group development. The first two group leaders should run a pre-group session in which they screen members for possible inclusion in the group and address ground rules and expectations. After this role-play is complete, the second group of co-leaders and group members should role-play the initial stage (forming) of a group. Then do the same for the transition stage (storming then norming), work stage (performing), and closure stage (adjourning) of the group. The rest of the class will view these role-plays and respond to the following questions:
1. How open are the group members in each stage?
2. Describe the amount of confrontation among members during each stage.
3. Describe the amount of confrontation with the group leader in each stage.
4. In each stage, compare the amount of discussion about "self" and discussion about "other."
5. Describe the amount of discussion of feelings as compared to the discussion of action-oriented self-help statements during each stage.
6. What kinds of counseling skills are used predominantly in each stage?

B. Watching a Video of a Group
Instead of role-playing a group as in Exercise A, view a videotape of a group and respond to the same questions above.

C. Shortened Version of Exercises A and B
Reflect on the questions in Exercise A and for each question, write down the kinds of expected behaviors you might see. Share your answers with the class.

X. Group Therapy
1. After completing Exercise IX, describe how the responses may have been different if this were a therapy group as opposed to a counseling group.
2. Discuss the differences, if any, that you believe exist between group counseling and group therapy.

XI. Rules of Group Behavior
Compare and contrast self-help groups, task groups, psychoeducational groups, counseling groups, and therapy groups on the items listed below:
1. What are the limits of confidentiality?
2. Can members socialize outside the group?
3. Can members date outside the group?
4. What expectations do you have concerning attendance in group sessions?
5. What expectations do you have concerning self-disclosure of members?
6. What are the repercussions and limits of physical acting out during group sessions?
7. Are there expectations concerning the types of things to be discussed during group sessions?
8. What expectations have you for member punctuality and whether members stay for the whole group meeting?

9. What expectations do you have concerning how members communicate during group sessions?
10. What is your responsibility to a member and to the group should you suspect that a specific member might cause harm to him- or herself or others?
11. How reasonable is it for you to be able to run each of the four groups noted in different settings (e.g., k-12 schools, colleges, agencies)?

XII. Comparison of Psychoeducational, Counseling, and Therapy Groups

Place each of the terms below where you think it should go in Figure 7.1 for each of the three kinds of groups listed. For instance, the word "Past" could be placed next to "Low" for psychoeducational groups, "Medium" for counseling groups, and "High" for psychotherapy groups. In class, your instructor should place Figure 7.1 on the board while students share their responses. Compare and discuss your responses.

Terms: Wellness, past, prevention, education, insight, group process, group dynamics, self-disclosure of members, pathology, change, conscious issues, unconscious issues, short-term, long-term

XIII. Use of Theory in Group Work
A. Theory-Specific Counseling and Therapy Groups

Individually or in small groups, take one of the theoretical orientations listed below (or another of your choosing), and describe how it could be applied to group work. Use the questions below to stimulate your responses. If time allows, do additional theories.

Theories: Psychoanalytic, Jungian, Adlerian, existential, person-centered, Gestalt, behavior therapy, cognitive therapy, reality therapy, narrative therapy, solution-focused behavior therapy

1. How is the view of human nature adapted to a group counseling/therapy approach?
2. Does the view of human nature dictate whether the approach will be short term, of medium length, or long term?
3. If the view of human nature lends itself to long-term counseling, can it somehow be adapted to group counseling that is generally of shorter duration?
4. Describe how the therapeutic relationship is adapted to a group approach.
5. What techniques from the theory seems most adaptable to a group approach? How?
6. Is it possible to draw from the different theories and develop an eclectic/integrative approach to group counseling/therapy? How would you do that?

B. Eclectic or Integrative Approach to Group Work

Your instructor will first break the class into small groups to ensure that each group has students who worked on a variety of different theories from "A." Discuss how you might be able to develop an eclectic approach to group work by borrowing various views of human nature and techniques from the different theories. Address each of the following:

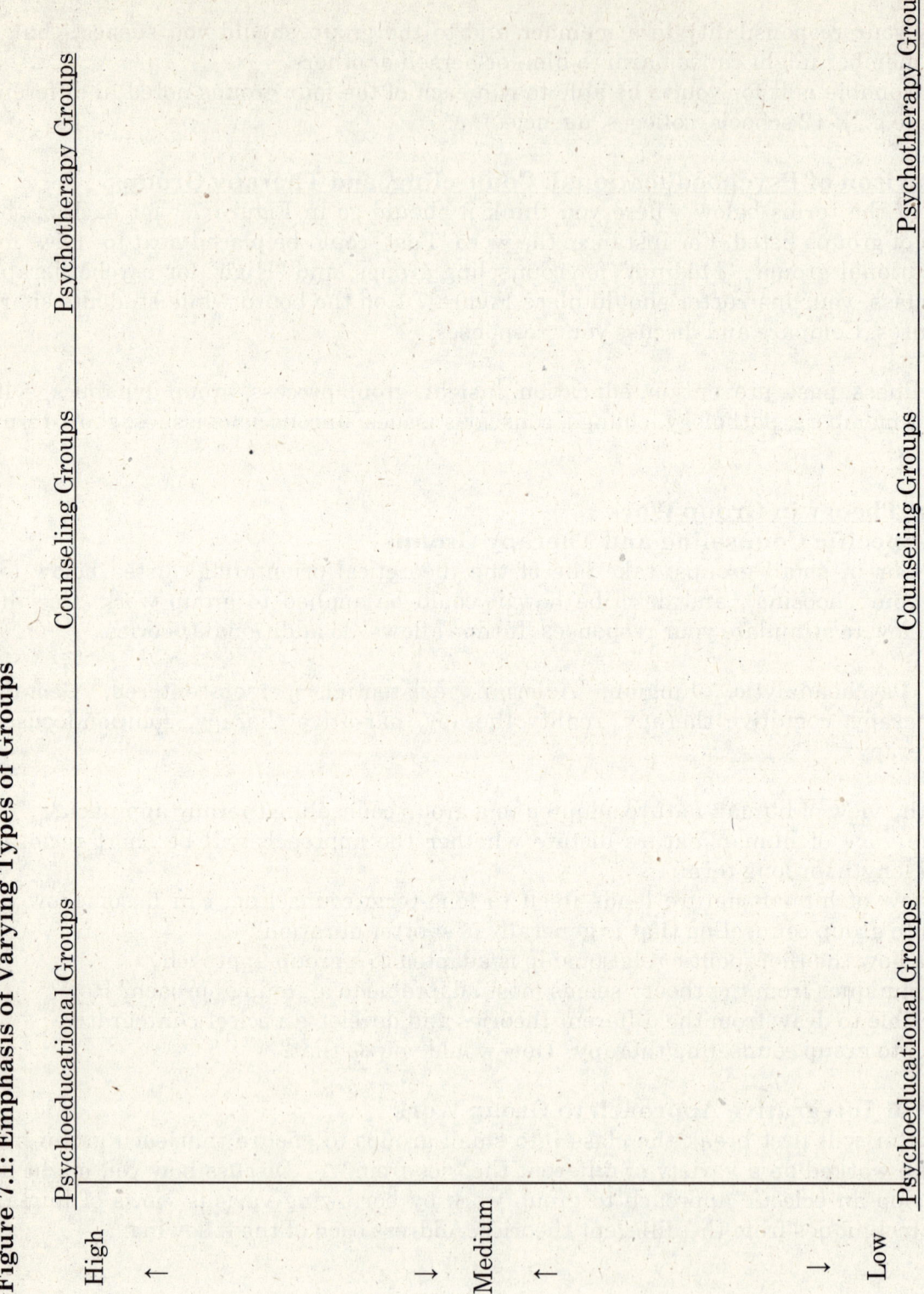

Figure 7.1: Emphasis of Varying Types of Groups

1. Explain your view of human nature, and show how you borrowed from different theoretical approaches.
2. Describe the therapeutic relationship, and show how you drew from the different approaches.
3. List your techniques, and note the theoretical approach the technique originated from.
4. Describe the typical course of treatment.

XIV. Experiential Group Learning

Your instructor will have the class break into triads. In these triads, you should discuss how you have had some group experience that has brought forth one or more of the factors described below (see Yalom & Leszcz 2005). Be forewarned that what you share in your triad may be shared with the class. When triads have finished sharing, your instructor will list the 12 factors on the board and ask for you to share some of the more interesting stories you heard from your classmates relative to each of these factors. Then, your instructor should lead a discussion about how all the factors are crucial to group process.

1. *Altruism*: Giving to others, helping others.
2. *Group cohesiveness:* Feeling a self of belonging and togetherness.
3. *Universality:* Gaining the sense that others go through similar experiences and problems.
4. *Interpersonal learning:* Learning, through feedback from others, how one interacts.
5. *Guidance:* Getting advice and direction from others.
6. *Catharsis:* Having an emotional release.
7. *Identification:* Taking on the behaviors of a person because one admires him or her.
8. *Family reenactment:* Gaining greater understanding about one's family of origin by recognizing patterns and gaining insight about those patterns.
9. *Self-understanding:* Gaining a deeper insight and broader awareness of self.
10. *Instillation of hope:* Feeling encouraged about the future; having a sense of problem amelioration.
11. *Existential factors:* Gaining an understanding that life brings with it painful and joyful experiences; learning about the natural rhythms of living.

* This exercise was adapted from material by Dr. Gerald Sklare, University of Louisville. His contribution is greatly appreciated.

XV. Multicultural and Social Justice Issues in Group Work

The diversity principles of the Association of Specialists in Group Work (ASGW) speak to the knowledge, skills, attitudes, and beliefs that all diversity-competent group workers should have. After reviewing the principles at http://www.asgw.org/diversity.htm, discuss the following questions in small groups or as a class:

1. How do you think issues of diversity get played out in groups?
2. What special knowledge as a leader do you need to have to be effective in running groups with members who are from different culture/ethnic background than you and/or the other group member?
3. How do groups represent a microcosm of society?
4. What positive or negative experiences in groups have you had that were a product of your ethnic or cultural background

XVI. Ethical, Legal, and Professional Vignettes

(The ACA's code is at www.counseling.org under "Resources"). In responding to the following, consider referring to the ACA's code.

1. A group leader decides to run a substance-abuse group for individuals in recovery. After the group had met for a few weeks, a member states that he is not getting anything out of the group and is going to quit. The group leader says to him that he should consider spending more time in the group to understand some of the underlying reasons why he wants to drop out. At this point, the other group members start pressuring him to stay, and tell him he is a "loser," a "user," and that he's going to find himself dead from drug use. The group leader allows the verbal barrage to continue until the group member breaks down and says, "Okay, I'll stay." Is this ethical? Professional?

2. After setting a ground rule that group members cannot date, a group leader finds that two members are seeing one another. He immediately throws them out of the group. Is this ethical? Is this professional? How should the group leader process this issue with the other group members?

3. Despite the fact that a group leader stresses the importance of confidentiality, the leader discovers that some intimate information about a group member has been leaked by another member. The group member asks who in the group broke confidentiality, and no one answers. Therefore, the leader decides to meet individually with each member in an attempt to find out who broke confidentiality. Is this ethical? Professional? Do you have other ideas about what the leader should do?

4. A group member shares that he has committed a robbery. Subsequently, he is arrested by the police, and the group leader is subpoenaed to testify about what he heard in the group. The leader is not a licensed counselor. Can he be forced to testify? Is it ethical for him to testify?

5. Use vignette 4, but this time assume the group leader is licensed. Under what circumstances, if any, can he be made to testify?

6. Use vignette 4, but this time, instead of having the leader subpoenaed, the group members are subpoenaed. Can they be forced to testify?

7. After having met for a few weeks, a group leader decides to incorporate some experiential activities that focus on intense expression of feelings. A couple of the members tell him that based on the informed consent statement they had read prior to starting the group, this was not expected. Is the group leader acting ethically? Professionally?

8. A school counselor who is running a short-term counseling group on self-esteem is called by a parent who is upset that his child was placed in a group without parental consent. Are the counselor's actions ethical? Professional? Legal?

9. In the course of a college therapy group, a student reveals that he committed date rape when out with a college friend. The counselor does not act on this knowledge because he wants to protect the confidentiality of the student. Is this ethical? Professional? Legal?

10. A group member who is involved in the same group as in vignette 9 decides to go to the police with the information he has heard. The police subsequently pick up the student and interrogated him. The student decides to sue the counselor for not securing confidentiality in the group. Can he sue? Is he justified?

11. After meeting for one year, a group ends. The group decides to go out for a dinner and invites the leader. The leader decides to go. Is this ethical? Professional?

12. A high school counselor decides to run a short-term counseling group for at-risk students. While running the group, some of the girls ask him where they can get information on birth control. He gives them the phone number and address of the local Planned Parenthood agency. Is this ethical? Legal?
13. In the course of running a self-esteem group for tenth graders, you learn that one of the group members is pregnant. She says she wants to have an abortion. You tell the group members to keep this information confidential and do not inform the girl's parents. Is this ethical? Professional? Legal?
14. When learning that a girl in a group is pregnant and wants to have an abortion, a group leader encourages the girl to consider keeping the child or adopting it out. Other group members concur, and the group leader gets them to promise that they will support her. Is this ethical? Professional? Legal?
15. A friend of yours is running a group that focuses on understanding dreams. He invites you to join. Upon hearing this, you ask him if he thinks that your being in the group constitutes a dual relationship. He states that this is not a therapy group, but a psychoeducational group, and that there would be no difficulty. Do you agree with his assessment? Is this ethical? Professional?
16. The same counselor as in vignette 15 is aware that some insurance companies pay for group counseling. He therefore decides to submit the names of his dream group clients to their respective insurance companies, stating that they are participating in group counseling. Is he acting ethically? Professionally? Legally?

CHAPTER 8

CONSULTATION AND SUPERVISION

PART I: CONSULTATION

I. Examples of Consultation

Consultation is

> When a professional (the consultant), who has specialized expertise, meets with one or more other professionals to improve the professionals' work with current or potential clients.

With the above definition in mind, and keeping in mind that consultation is not counseling, give examples of how a counselor could be a consultant in the following settings. Share your responses in class.

Consultation in Agencies:

Consultation in Schools:

Consultation in Colleges:

Consultation in Business and Industry:

II. Implementation of Different Types of Consultation

After reviewing the types of consultant- and system-centered types of consultation listed, describe some ways in which you might apply each in a school, agency, college, or other setting of your choice.

Consultant-Centered Consultation

1. *Expert consultation model.* Here, the consultant is specifically brought into an organization because of his or her expertise in a specific area and asked to use this knowledge to provide solutions to specific problems (Schein, 1969, 1999).
2. *Prescriptive consultation model (doctor-patient mode).* Here the consultant collects information, diagnoses the problem, and makes recommendations to the consultee on how to solve the problem (Dougherty, 2009; Schein, 1969, 1999).
3. *Trainer/educator consultation model.* Often used in what has come to be known as "staff development" (Dougherty, 2009), in this mode, the consultant is hired to come into a system and teach or train the staff.

System-Centered Consultation

1. *Collaborative consultation model.* In this type of consultation, a partnership develops in which the consultant offers expertise but also relies on the expertise of individuals in the system to offer input into problems and solutions (Idol, Nevin, & Paolucci-Whitcomb, 2000). This shared expertise model tends to focus on joint decision-making (Kampwirth, 2006).
2. *Facilitative consultation model.* Here, the consultant plays a facilitative role by helping individuals within the system communicate with one another, understand each other, and resolve conflicts among themselves (Dougherty, 2009; Rubenstein, 1973; Schein, 1999).
3. *Process-oriented consultation model.* This consultant either believes that he or she does not have the answer or withholds expertise with the belief that the most effective resolution, resulting in the highest self-esteem and sense of ownership of the problem, would be for the system members to find their own solution. The consultant has faith that system members can change if the consultant is able to develop a trusting environment in which such change can occur (Dougherty, 2009; Schein, 1969, 1999).

III. Consultation at a Mental Health Center

First, your instructor should ask you to do Exercise A and/or B that follows. Then, after reviewing the types of consultation in Exercise II, show how you would assist the agency described in Exercise A or B through the following stages of consultation: Stage 1: pre-entry; Stage 2: entry, problem exploration, and contracting; Stage 3: information gathering, problem confirmation, and goal setting; Stage 4: solution searching and intervention selection; Stage 5: evaluation; and Stage 6: termination. In your response, show how the consultative process is systemic and how it is developmental (deals with developmental issues and is preventive).

A. Operationalizing Styles of Consultation

After reading the description of the agency in Appendix F, describe how you would operationalize one or more specific styles of consultation noted in Exercise II, and then describe how you might use that approach to facilitate change in the system.

B. Role-Playing Consultation

After reading the description of the agency in Appendix F, your instructor will ask for volunteers to be directors, outpatient counselors, inpatient counselors, day treatment counselors, clerical staff, and two consultants, both of whom practice one of the types of consultation listed in Exercise II. The rest of the class can act as observers, giving feedback about the efficacy of the approach taken.

IV. Consultation at a School

A. Consultation to Change School Atmosphere

After reviewing the types of consultation in Exercise II, show how you would assist the school described in Box 8.1 through the following stages of consultation: Stage 1: pre-entry; Stage 2: entry, problem exploration, and contracting; Stage 3: information gathering, problem confirmation, and goal setting; Stage 4: solution searching and intervention selection; Stage 5: evaluation; and Stage 6: termination. In your response, show how the consultative process is systemic, preventive, and developmental.

> **Box 8.1: Consultation in a School**
>
> You're one of two middle school counselors in a school of 50 teachers. The principal has approached you because she believes that too many teachers are critical of students in their classrooms. She even describes a few teachers as being verbally abusive in the class. She also reveals to you that a number of parents have been complaining about the attitude of some of the teachers. In addition, she notes that the clerical staff seems to have a negative attitude when teachers ask for assistance and when answering the phone. She would like you to deal with the whole problem.

B. Operationalizing Different Kinds of School Consultation

Referring back to the different kinds of consultation in Exercise II, explain how you might implement a consultation model for each of the examples below:

1. Assisting teachers in understanding the psychological, sociological, and learning needs of students

2. Assisting teachers in classroom management techniques

3. Assisting teachers, administrators, and parents in understanding the developmental needs of children and how they might affect learning

4. Meeting with students to help them understand developmental concerns, peer relationship issues, personal concerns, and other issues

5. Meeting with other professionals in the community concerning the needs of a particular student with whom the counselor is working

6. Meeting with parents, teachers, and specialists regarding the individual education plan of a special needs student

7. Assisting students in becoming peer counselors and conflict mediators

8. Assisting school staff in setting up a school environment that is conducive to learning for individuals from all cultures

9. Offering organizational consulting skills to assist administrators and others in the efficient running of the school

10. Offering administrators, parents, teachers, and students assistance in understanding the purpose of assessment instruments and how to interpret their results

C. School and Agency Consultation

Contact a school counselor who is working with a student who is also being seen at an agency with which the school counselor has contact. Without asking for information about the student, interview the school counselor and the agency helper about their collaboration:

1. How did the working relationship start?

2. How is the working arrangement viewed by each (e.g., collaborative, hierarchical, competitive, etc.)?

3. Does each helper have a slightly different view of the relationship?

4. How is the partnership "successful"?

5. What are some of the barriers to the partnership?

6. How might you change this arrangement if you were the school counselor?

* Exercise C was adapted from material by Garry Gleckel, Keene State College. His contribution is greatly appreciated.

V. Consultation at a University

A. Consultation for Cross-Cultural Tension

After reviewing the types of consultation in Exercise II, show how you would assist the university described in Box 8.2 through the following stages of consultation: Stage 1: pre-entry; Stage 2: entry, problem exploration, and contracting; Stage 3: information gathering, problem confirmation, and goal setting; Stage 4: solution searching and intervention selection; Stage 5: evaluation; and Stage 6: termination. In your response, show how the consultative process is systemic and how it is developmental (deals with developmental issues and is preventive).

Box 8.2: Consultation at a University

You work at a university counseling center, and the director has approached the counseling staff because the president of the university is concerned about cross-cultural tensions throughout the university. The director describes to the staff incidences of harassment among students from different cultures and concerns about lack of knowledge as well as insensitivity to different cultures among administrators, faculty, and staff at the college. The director would like the counseling staff to develop and implement a consultation plan that deals with this problem. The director is hoping that the result of this consultation would be the development of goals that the university can begin to implement.

B. A Model of College Consultation

Using the model below in Figure 8.1, see if you can briefly describe an individual, group, or organizational training program for each of the audiences listed (students, faculty, staff, and administrators). For each audience, come up with at least one training program (education/training, program wide, doctor-patient, or process oriented). For instance, one type of process model would include having faculty get together in small groups, run by a facilitator, to discuss students who "act out" in class.

Figure 8.1: College Counseling Supervision Model

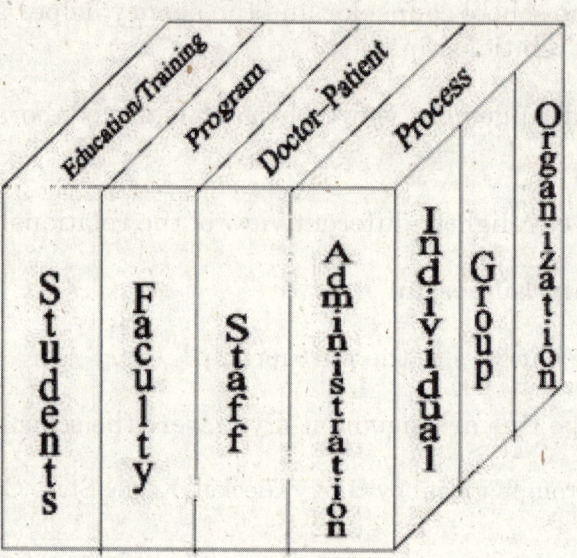

From: Cooper, S. (2003). College counseling centers as internal organizational consultants to universities. *Consulting Psychology Journal: Practice and Research*, 55(4), p. 234.

VI. Utilizing Counseling Theory in Consultation

Over the years, various counseling theories have been employed when providing consultation. Using Appendix F, Box 8.1, and/or Box 8.2, explore which counseling approaches you think would best be used with consultation process given (e.g., psychodynamic, existential-humanistic, cognitive-behavioral, post-modern, etc.). Discuss the following items in groups of two to five:

1. What are advantages or disadvantages to using counseling approaches during consultation?

2. What type(s) of consultation is most conducive to applying counseling approaches? Why?

3. How might consultation employing a specific counseling approach differ dependent upon the setting?

4. Are some counseling approaches or theories more applicable to consultation than others?

* This exercise was adapted from material by Dr. Jeffrey Warren, North Carolina State University. His contribution is greatly appreciated.

PART II: SUPERVISION

VII. Consultation and Supervision: Similarities and Differences
Using the definition of consultation in Exercise I, show how supervision is a type of consultation. Then describe how it differs from most forms of consultation.

VIII. Supervision: A Systemic Process
1. List and describe all the individuals and systems that may be affected by supervision.
2. Describe a supervisee's responsibility toward his or her (a) clients, (b) immediate family of clients, (c) friends and extended family of client, (d) acquaintances of clients, and (e) systems affected by clients (e.g., a client's workplace)?
3. Describe the supervisor's responsibility toward the people listed in item 2.

IX. Characteristics of the Effective Supervisor
In small groups or as a class, make a list of personality characteristics you would like to see in a supervisor. Under what circumstances would each of them be effective?

X. Parallel Process
Parallel process occurs in the supervisory relationship when the client/counselor relationship is mimicked in the supervisor/supervisee relationship. This generally occurs when the counselor unconsciously takes on the traits of the client, which are repeated in the supervisory relationship (e.g., taking on the client's anxiety and repeating it in supervision). With this in mind, read the vignette in Box 8.2 and discuss, in small groups, reasons why this parallel process could occur in this situation. Then discuss how the supervisor could use his or her skills to avoid the same parallel process in supervision and to help Juan work effectively work with Suzanne.

Box 8.2: Parallel Process
Juan is in supervision with Carla. One of his clients, Suzanne, is having panic attacks. Suzanne has two children, works full time, and is in graduate school. Her marriage is "rocky." Economically, she cannot back off from work, and her dream is to finish her graduate degree. She comes to Juan pleading for help, noting that throughout the day she has panic attacks and at night she has difficulty sleeping. She is worried about being able to tend to her children and her studies because of her state of mind. A psychiatric consult and subsequent medication has resulted in little relief. She looks at Juan and says, "Please, you've got to help me—what should I do?" Juan is stymied, and at his first opportunity, discusses Suzanne's situation with Carla. Juan notes to Carla, "You know, since I've been working with Suzanne I am filled with anxiety. I feel inadequate because I can't find a solution for her. I am thinking about her situation all the time, cannot stop obsessing about it, and I am having trouble sleeping because I am worrying about her. It's even affecting my relationship with my partner.

XI. Styles of Supervision
A. Developmental Supervision
Developmental models, such as the Integrated Developmental Model (IDM) of Stoltenberg and colleagues (Stoletenberg, 2005; Stoltenberg & Delworth, 1987; Stoltenberg, McNeill, &

Delworth, 1998), view supervision through a series of stages during which the supervisee will pass as he or she obtains supervision (Borders & Brown, 2005). Therefore, the supervisor can rely on a certain amount of predictable growth as well as resistance, depending on the stage of the supervisee. Using Table 8.1, explain changes in each of the attributes listed as a function of stage of supervision (beginning, middle, and late stage).

Table 8.1: Changes in Supervisee During Supervision

	Beginning Stage	Middle Stage	Late Stage
Knowledge about Counseling			
Knowledge about Self in Relation to Client			
Motivation for Supervision			
Dependency to Supervisor			
Resistance toward the Supervision Process			
Increase Knowledge and Sensitivity Toward Diversity			

B. Psychotherapy-Based Models of Supervision

Psychotherapy-based models allow the supervisor to either model or teach a specific theoretical orientation to the supervisee. For instance, a behavioral supervisor could model a behavioral approach by identifying problems in supervision, collaboratively setting goals to work on, and then using techniques to reach those goals. Or, using the teaching approach, a psychoanalytic supervisor might offer suggestions on how to use a specific psychoanalytic technique with a client. With this in mind, pick a counseling theory of your choice and describe the following:

1. The major tenets of the theory that would be applied to the supervisory process.
2. How you would model such a theory in supervision.
3. How you would teach such a technique in supervision.
4. Whether you think "modeling" or "teaching" works better for the particularly counseling theory that you chose to use in supervision.

C. Integrated Models of Supervision

Sometimes called meta-theory models, integrative models are not theory specific and can be used regardless of the theoretical approach of the supervisee. Items 1 and 2 offer two examples of integrated models.

1. *Bernard's Discriminant Model.* This model views the supervisor as a teacher, counselor, and consultant who focuses on specific interventions, case conceptualization, and personalization (personal issues) of the supervisee. Using the example in Box 8.2 of

Exercise X, in small groups, show how the supervise might use each of his or her role for each focus of supervision. Write your answers in Table 8.2.

Table 8.2: Roles and Foci of Discriminant Model

Focus of Supervision	Roles of Supervisor		
	Teacher ↓	Counselor ↓	Consultant ↓
Intervention→			
Conceptualization→			
Personalization→			

2. *Interpersonal Process Recall (IPR).* This model relies on the trainee to uncover his or her strengths and weaknesses by having the supervisor and trainee meet together and listen or view an audio or video recording of the trainee (Kagan, 1980; Kagan & Kagan, 1997). The trainee, supervisor, or both can control the recording, starting and stopping it when it is believed that there is an important moment in counseling. The supervisor's role is to attend accurately to the feelings and thoughts of the supervisee, and when appropriate, ask leading questions to deepen the session. Typical questions asked in this kind of supervision include the following:
   1. What do you wish you had said to him or her?
   2. How do you think he or she would have reacted if you had said that?
   3. What would have been the risk in saying what you wanted to say?
   4. If you had the chance now, how might you tell him or her what you are thinking and feeling?
   5. Were there any other thoughts going through your mind?
   6. How did you want the other person to perceive you?
   7. Were those feelings located physically in some part of your body?
   8. Were you aware of any feelings? Does that feeling have any special meaning for you?
   9. What did you want him or her to tell you?
   10. What did you think he or she wanted from you?
   11. Did he or she remind you of anyone in your life? (Cashwell, 1994, p. 2)

Using this model, break up into triads and role-play an IPR session. One person will play the supervisor and one person will play the supervisee who is discussing a client. The third person is an observer who can give critical feedback at any point during the process.

XII. Supervision of Graduate Students

As you go through graduate school, you will undoubtedly obtain many opportunities to attain supervision. For instance, supervision is likely to occur in an early counseling skills class where you will receive peer supervision and/or supervision by a faculty member, in a practicum by a faculty member and/or site supervisor, and in an internship by a faculty member and/or site supervisor. Considering each of these opportunities for supervision, answer the following:

1. At this point in your studies, of the three types of supervision listed in Exercise XI, with which type would you feel most comfortable? Why?
2. Of the different types of supervision listed in Exercise XI, which do you believe would be most useful for students in a skills class, practicum class, and internship class? Why?
3. How might developmental differences make a difference in the kind of supervision applied to a graduate student?
4. How might personality differences make a difference in the kind of supervision applied to a graduate student?

XIII. Supervision in the Workplace

1. Explain the importance of supervision for a school counselor, agency counselor, private practitioner, college counselor, or other kind of counselor.
2. Discuss reasons why supervision is sometimes ineffective at the workplace.
3. What kind of supervision do you believe would work best in a school, agency, private practice setting, college counseling center, or other counseling settings?

XIV Ethical, Legal, and Professional Vignettes

(The ACA's code is at www.counseling.org under "Resources"). In responding to the following, consider referring to the ACA's code.

A. Consultation

1. A consultant who was called in to deal with systemic problems in an agency is asked privately by the administrator of the agency to let him know if any staff members seem to be having serious emotional problems. The administrator would like to assist staff in finding help for their problems. The consultant complies and tells the administrator of a secretary and a counselor who are under particular emotional stress. Is this ethical? Professional?
2. At a substance-abuse agency, a consultant who was called in to deal with systemic problems in the agency is privately asked by the administrator of the agency to let her know if any staff are using drugs. The administrator plans on letting go any staff who are using. The consultant complies and lets the administrator know that one staff person is smoking marijuana. The administrator fires this person. Has the administrator acted ethically? Professionally? Legally? Has the consultant acted ethically? Professionally? Legally?
3. A consultant is told by a number of African-American staff that he can never understand their situation because he is White. What should the consultant do?
4. A school counselor is asked by the principal of his school to consult with teachers and uncover any feelings of discontent they may be having with the administrators. Upon meeting with teachers, the school counselor becomes aware that they see her as "siding with" the administrators. What should she do?

5. Using the same example as in vignette 4, does the fact that the consultant already works in the school constitute an ethical violation of "dual relationships"?
6. While consulting at a university with faculty, a consultant discovers that a staff member is suicidal. The consultant attempts to refer the staff person to counseling, but he refuses. The consultant decides to try and have the staff member committed to a psychiatric unit. Has the consultant acted ethically? Professionally? Legally?
7. A counselor is hired by a business to consult with them regarding sexual harassment at the workplace. The counselor knows little about consultation theory, but much about sexual harassment. She decides to read some books on consultation and proceeds to consult. Has she acted ethically? Professionally?
8. A counselor is hired by a business to meet with employees in an attempt to discover if employees are lax on the job. The counselor tells the employees that she is looking at "overall job performance" of the business. Does the counselor's stretching of the truth constitute lack of informed consent? Is this an ethical violation? Is this professional?

B. Supervision

9. After meeting with a supervisee, a supervisor believes that one of the supervisee's clients is in danger of harming herself. The supervisee believes that the client is not at risk and decides not to take any action, despite requests by the supervisor. The supervisor decides to contact the client herself and makes arrangements to have her committed to a psychiatric unit. Has the supervisee acted ethically? Professionally? Has the supervisor acted ethically? Professionally?
10. In offering a professional disclosure statement to clients, a counselor fails to tell clients that she is being supervised. Is this ethical? Professional?
11. A supervisor believes that a counselor is doing harm to a client and insists that the counselor change his approach to working with the client. The counselor argues that he believes he is helping the client. The supervisor tells the counselor to either change his approach or be fired. Has the supervisee acted ethically? Professionally? Has the supervisor acted ethically? Professionally?
12. A supervisor becomes attracted to his supervisee, and they begin to increasingly have more social contact. Has the supervisee acted ethically? Professionally? Has the supervisor acted ethically? Professionally?
13. Using the example in vignette 12, but this time the supervisor and supervisee engage in a sexual relationship. Has the supervisee acted ethically? Professionally? Has the supervisor acted ethically? Professionally?
14. A supervisee who had been involved in a sexual relationship with her supervisee later believes that the relationship constitutes sexual harassment. Could she be correct? If this is sexual harassment, what can she do?
15. A supervisee believes that her supervisor is incompetent and giving her poor supervision. She decides to report him to the state licensing board. Has she acted ethically? Professionally? Is there anything else she could have done?
16. A supervisor routinely endorses his supervisees for licensure as school counselors and as licensed professional counselors, despite the fact that he believes some of his supervisee are "too green to be out there." Has this supervisor acted ethically? Professionally?
17. Despite not having any training in supervision, a supervisor oversees the supervision of a number of counselors. Is this ethical? Professional?

CHAPTER 9

HUMAN DEVELOPMENT: NORMAL AND ABNORMAL

I. Who Are You?

A. Personality Characteristics

Below is a list of words, some of which are likely to describe you. Although we tend to show all of these traits at different times, for the purposes of this exercise, within each pair of words, circle the one that you are more like. Then, reflect on how you think you may have acquired these characteristics.

Introverted/Extroverted	Slow/Fast
Angry/Serene	Assertive/Passive
Focused/Scattered	In Touch/Out of Touch
Depressed/Happy	Abstract/Concrete
Anxious/Calm	Desperate/Hopeful
Dominant/Submissive	Fastidious/Sloppy
Skinny/Obese	Winner/Loser
Healthy/Sickly	Tolerant/Intolerant
Responsible/Irresponsible	Flexible/Rigid
High Self-Concept/Low Self-Concept	Dominant/Submissive
Internal Locus of Control/External Locus of Control	

B. Comparing Yourself to Others

Your instructor will pick three pairs of words from the list in Exercise A. Considering all possible combinations of words that could be formed from those three pairs of words, students should next join up with other students who have the same combination of words. For instance, if the instructor were to choose introverted/extroverted, slow/fast, and angry/serene, the following groups would be formed:

introverted/slow/angry	introverted/slow/serene	introverted fast/angry
introverted/fast/serene	extroverted/slow/angry	extroverted/slow/serene
extroverted/fast/angry	extroverted/fast/serene	

Now, in your groups, discuss how your qualities were acquired. Refer to specific personality theories whenever possible. For instance, is a person introverted because of genetics, because he or she learned through modeling to be introverted, because of how he or she experienced the psychosexual stages of development, or for some other reasons?

II. Reflecting on Your Personality Development

From a psychodynamic, humanistic, learning theory, post-modern (social constructionist), or other personality development perspective, describe the following:
1. How does each perspective explain characteristics of your personality?
2. In explaining your personality development from the differing perspectives, what commonalities do you see between the varying theories?
3. In explaining your personality development from the differing perspectives, what differences do you see between the varying theories?

III. Defense Mechanisms
A. Reviewing Defense Mechanisms
Provide an example of each of the following defense common mechanisms:

Repression	Denial	Projection
Displacement	Rationalization	Regression
Introjection	Compensation	Reaction formation
Intellectualization	Identification	Sublimation

B. Understanding Our Defense Mechanisms
After completing Exercise A, reflect on how you use one or more of the defense mechanisms above. Can you identify other defense mechanisms you might use?

C. Developing Defense Mechanisms
Using psychodynamic, humanistic, learning theory, post-modern, or another approach of your choice, describe how you may have developed the above defense mechanisms.

IV. Examining Your Development
A. Acknowledging Your Place in History
Gilleard & Higgs (2007) assert that development is affected by one's generational cohort. Without accurate representation of the needs, resources, and vulnerabilities of an individual within his or her historical context, it is impossible to accurately assess the individual's developmental problems, resources, and coping skills. For the following activity, the class will be divided by dates of birth before 1959, 1960-1969, 1970-1985, 1986, and beyond. Each group will identify what they recall about the following when they were between the ages of 5 and 15. List as many as you can in each of these categories:
1. What was the social, economic, and political climate?
2. What were the advances of medicine, science, and technology?
3. What were family patterns and sexual values like?
4. What do you recall about education and recreation, games, and toys?
5. Were there any issues that polarized the country?
6. Who were the icons, heroes, and entertainers?
7. What was representative of art and music?
8. What slogans, sayings, lyrics, and slang do remember?

After each group has presented their lists to the rest of the class, discuss how a difference in generational age cohort might influence one's understanding of an individual client, a group, or a family.[1]

B. Erickson Lifespan Theory
Review Table 9.1 of Erickson's theory (Erickson, 1963, 1980, 1982) and respond to the following questions:
1. After reading each stage, with which stage or stages might you have struggled?
2. How did struggling in that stage affect the development of your particular virtue?
3. How did struggling in a particular stage affect the stages that follow?
4. What have you done to resolve some of the issues of that stage?

---

[1] This exercise was adapted from material by Dr. Nicki Nance, Webster University, Ocala Metropolitan Campus. Her contribution is greatly appreciated.

Table 9.1: Erikson's Psychosocial Stages of Development

Stage	Name of Stage with Ages	Virtue of Stage	Description of Stage
1	Trust vs. Mistrust (Birth-1)	Hope	In this stage, the infant is building a sense of trust or mistrust that can be facilitated by significant others' ability to provide a sense of psychological safety to the infant.
2	Autonomy vs. Shame and Doubt (1-2)	Will	Here, the toddler explores the environment and is beginning to gain control over his or her body. Significant others can either promote or inhibit the child's newfound abilities and facilitate the development of autonomy or shame and doubt.
3	Initiative vs. Guilt (3-5)	Purpose	As physical and intellectual growth continues and exploration of the environment increases, a sense of initiative or guilt can be developed by significant others who are either encouraging or discouraging of the child's physical and intellectual curiosity.
4	Industry vs. Inferiority (6-11)	Competence	An increased sense of what the child is good at, especially relative to his or her peers, can either be reinforced or negated by significant others (e.g., parents, teachers, peers) leading to feeling worthwhile, or discouraged by others, which leads to feeling inferior.
5	Identity vs. Role Confusion (Adolescence)	Fidelity	Positive role models and experiences can lead to increased understanding of temperament, values, interests, and abilities that define one's sense of self. Negative role models and limited experiences will lead to role confusion.
6	Intimacy vs. Isolation (Early Adulthood)	Love	A good sense of self and self-understanding lead to the ability to form intimate relationships that are highlighted by mutually supporting relationships that encourage individuality with interdependency. Otherwise, the young adult feels isolated.
7	Generativity vs. Stagnation (Middle Adulthood)	Caring	Healthy development in this stage is highlighted by concern for others and for future generations. This individual is able to maintain a productive and responsible lifestyle and can find meaning through work, volunteerism, parenting, and/or community activities. Otherwise, the adult feels stagnant.
8	Ego Integrity vs. Despair (Later Life)	Wisdom	The older adult who examines his or her life either feels a sense of fulfillment or despair. Successfully mastering the developmental tasks from the preceding stages will lead to a sense of integrity for the individual.

5. What can you do to resolve some of the issues in that stage?
6. What can you do to assure seamless movement through the stages that will follow in your life?

C. Moral Development (Kohlberg and Gilligan)

Lawrence Kolbherg (1969, 1984) and Carol Gilligan (1982) have both written about moral development of children with somewhat slightly different views. Gilligan was concerned that Kohlberg did not fully understand the moral development of girls and women. Table 9.2 gives a very brief description of the stages as presented by Kohlberg and Gilligan. Read in your textbook more about these different ways of viewing moral development and respond to the following dilemma—one from Kohblerg's perspective and one from Gilligan's:

> Jaime is working at a counseling practice and wants to become a partner. One of the current partners tells Jaime that if Jaime works very hard and "does the right thing," she can do quite well in the office, and in a few years probably become a partner. At the next staff meeting, the same partner who had spoken with Jaime asks for everyone at the practice to see more clients, because overhead for the practice is rising. All the staff are already fully booked, working more than they should if they are to offer ethical counseling and not become burnt out. Jaime needs to decide how to respond to this somewhat outrageous proposal. Jaime realizes that promotion in the office is at stake.

1. Go through each of Kohlberg's stages, and in small groups, discuss how a person would respond.
2. Go through each of Gillgian's stages, and in small group, discuss how a person would respond.
3. Do you believe Kohlberg and Gilligan's differences are sex-based? That is, would men be more likely to respond as Kohlberg stated and would women be more likely to respond as Gilligan stated?

Table 9.2: Comparing Kohlberg and Gilligan

Kohlberg/ Gilligan Levels	Kohlberg	Gilligan
Preconventional	1. Punishment/reward. 2. Satisfy needs to gain reward (you get from me, I get from you).	Concern for survival.
Conventional	1. Social conformity/ approval of others. 2. Rules and laws to maintain order.	Caring for others. Sacrifice of self for others. Responsible to others.
Postconventional	1. Social contract/democratically arrived at. Rules that can be changed through a logical process. 2. Individual conscience.	Decision-making from an interdependent perspective. All that we choose affects everyone else.

D. Kegan's Interpersonal Model (*Subject-Object Theory*)

Robert Kegan (1982, 1984) believes our understanding of the world is based on how we construct reality through the lifespan. He states there are six stages of cognitive development (stages 0 to 5), with stages 2, 3, 4, and 5 representing ways in which adults view the world. Movement from a lower to higher stage necessitates letting go of the earlier stage. In small groups, read the brief definitions of the stages in Box 9.1 and respond to the following questions:

1. Identify which stage you are likely in.
2. Discuss what evidence you have to show that you are in this stage.
3. What can you do to facilitate movement to a higher stage?
4. What can your counseling program do to facilitate movement to a higher stage?

Box 9.1: Kegan's Stages*

Imperial stage: Stage 2 is marked by a narcissistic desire to get one's needs met. Here, the person will manipulate others in an effort to feel good. There is little or no empathy, and a sense of caring for others is usually just shown in an effort to meet one's own needs.

Interpersonal stage: In stage 3, relationships are primary and needs and wishes are met through the relationship. Symbolically, the interpersonal person lives by the following statements, "I am you, and you are me. I do not exist without you. You make me who I am." This stage is symbolized by dependency. Beginning empathy is shown because the person has a need to show the "other" person he or she cares.

Institutional stage. Stage 4 is where a sense of autonomy and self-authorship is acquired. Relationships are important but no longer essential as values and interests become important. The individual chooses a partner because the other person shares similar values; however, the person does not need the partner as in the interpersonal stage. Empathy is a choice that can be shown at appropriate times (e.g., the counseling relationship, with a partner).

Interindividual stage: Stage 5 is highlighted by mutuality in relationships; that is, the individual can share and learn from others in a nondependent way. Differences are tolerated and even encouraged at times. This self-reflective individual encourages feedback about self. Like the self-actualized person, here, there is respect for self and for all others, regardless of their stage. This person embodies empathy as a mode of living.

*Stage 0 = Incoporative stage, Stage 1 = Impulsive stage

E. Fowler's Faith Development

Fowler (1976, 1991, 1995, 2000) believes that faith is universal, inherent, and relates to how we make meaning. Faith is much broader than a singular examination of one's religious orientation and means that the atheist, agnostic, fundamentalist, and communist all have some faith experience, for faith is not dependent on a belief in God. In addition, faith includes unconscious motivations. Fowler identified seven stages (0-6) with minimal ages at which a person can enter a stage. In small groups, read the brief definitions in Box 9.2 of the four stages in which most adults find themselves.

1. Identify which stage you are likely in.

2. Discuss what evidence you have to show that you are in this stage.
3. What can you do to facilitate movement to a higher stage?
4. What can your counseling program do to facilitate movement to a higher stage?

Box 9.2: Fowler's Stages*

Stage 3, Synthetic-Conventional Faith (12 to 13): In this stage, the person is beginning to synthesize many viewpoints; however, he or she remains embedded within his or her social sphere, and faith reflects only those values within that sphere.

Stage 4, Individuative-Reflective Faith (18 to 19): In this stage, the person begins to develop a new meaning-making system through reflection and introspection and by examining different points of view. This relativistic individual now recognizes different types of faith experiences and may move toward a new experience.

Stage 5, Conjunctive Faith (30 to 32): In this stage, the individual is able to honor and affirm others who have different faith commitments while not denying his or her own faith. There is a newfound understanding of symbols and metaphors related to one's own faith tradition, as well as the faith traditions of others. There is openness to other points of view, a commitment to one's own point of view, and a sense of humility regarding all that is known.

Stage 6, Universalizing Faith (38 to 40): This stage involves acceptance of others, regardless of stage or faith tradition. Called *decentration from self*, in this stage, the person has the ability to fully understand the views of others. This individual experiences faith as universal, beyond ideological beliefs, and is able to embrace all others. This individual can integrate and synthesize beliefs from many disparate viewpoints into a unique faith experience.

*Stage 0 = Primal Faith; Stage 1 = Intuitive Projective Faith; Stage 2 = Mythic-Literal Faith

---

F. Other Developmental Theories

In addition to the theories you just examined, identify another developmental theory of your choice (e.g., Piaget, Levinson, Perry) and discuss the following questions:
1. Has your life paralleled some of the stages listed in the theory?
2. What specific developmental tasks have you faced relative to one or more of the theories listed?
3. How have prior developmental stages affected your current functioning? How do you think prior stages may affect your future functioning?

V. Comparison of Developmental Theories

Compare and contrast the developmental theories listed in Exercise IV. What do they have in common? How do they differ?

VI. Examining the Development of an Adult with a Developmental Disability

Box 9.3 describes Gloria. After reading about Gloria, describe her from the following perspectives:

1. Child development viewpoint (e.g., physical, cognitive, and moral development)
2. Personality development viewpoint (e.g., psychoanalytic, humanistic, learning perspective)
3. Lifespan development perspective (e.g., Erikson)
4. Constructive development (e.g., Kegan, Perry, Fowler)

BOX 9.3 Gloria

Gloria is a 53-year-old person who was born mildly mentally retarded and with cerebral palsy. Soon after her birth, her parents placed her in an institution for the developmentally disabled. She lived there until she was 31, at which time she was placed in a group home for the mentally retarded.

As a child, Gloria's language development was delayed. She could not speak in sentences until she was 4. She was not toilet trained until age 7. Although her parents would visit her periodically, her main caretakers were the social service workers at the institution. Gloria was schooled at the institution where she acquired the equivalent of a second-grade education. Gloria had few friends in the institution and was considered a loner. Despite working on socialization skills while in the institution, Gloria still prefers to be alone and spends much of her time painting. She has become a rather good artist, and many of her paintings are found in the institution and in the group home. Visitors often comment on the paintings and are generally surprised that a developmentally disabled person can paint so well. Gloria has a part-time job at a local art-supply store where she generally does menial work.

Although Gloria does have some friends at the group home and at the art-supply store, generally, when she spends much time with someone, she ends up having a temper tantrum. When this happens, she will usually withdraw, often to her painting. She blames other people for her anger.

Gloria is a rules follower. She feels very strongly about the list of rules on the bulletin board at her group home. She methodically reports people who break them. She always feels extremely guilty after having a temper tantrum, because she sees herself as breaking the rule "talk things out rather than get into a fight." In a similar vein, Gloria feels that laws in the country "are there for a purpose." For instance, at street crossings, she always stops at red lights and waits for the light to change.

Gloria has no sense of her future. She lives from day to day, and despite periods of depression, generally functions fairly adequately. She states she wants to get married, but her lack of socialization skills prevents her from having any meaningful relationships with men.

Overall, the human service professionals who have contact with Gloria describe her as a rigid, conscientious, talented person who has trouble maintaining relationships. They note that despite being in individual counseling and in a socialization support group, she has made little progress in maintaining satisfying relationships. Their feeling is that she probably will maintain her current level of functioning, and they see little hope for change.

VII. Counseling Gloria: A Developmental Perspective

If you were to counsel Gloria (Box 9.3), how might your knowledge of developmental theory affect your work with her?

VIII. Examining the Development of a Gifted Child

Box 9.4 describes Joe. After reading about him, describe him from the following perspectives.

1. Child development viewpoint (e.g., physical, cognitive, and moral development)
2. Personality development viewpoint (e.g., psychoanalytic, humanistic, learning perspective)
3. Lifespan development perspective (e.g., Erikson)
4. Constructive development (e.g., Kegan, Perry, Fowler)

Box 9.4: Joe

Joe is 13 years old and the only child, grandchild, and niece or nephew on his mother's side of the family. Joe's parents separated when his mother was 5 months pregnant with him. His parents, both of whom are highly educated, went through a tumultuous separation and divorce but now have a cordial relationship. Following his birth, his mother was distraught over the breakup of her marriage but subsequently has maintained a strong sense of self and high self-esteem. Following Joe's birth, his mother, who works full time, was fortunately able to afford a live-in nanny. This woman still lives with them and has been a significant help for the family and an additional source of comfort for Joe.

Joe's mother remarried when Joe was 10 and his father has been involved in a long-term relationship. Joe lives with his mother but spends every other weekend, some weekdays, and extended periods of time during the summer and holidays with his father. He seems to have a good relationship with both parents, his stepfather, and his father's girlfriend

Joe, who has always done well in school, currently attends a private school. He maintains very high grades and has a high IQ. Joe is at ease in relationships, as evidenced by his many friends and his ability to relate to people of all ages. He has many skills and is just beginning to examine those things that he is best at. He is just entering puberty, and girls are becoming more important to him. Overall, most people would describe Joe as a bright, personable, and thoughtful young man who is at ease with himself.

Although sometimes he may appear a little "spoiled," he generally is thoughtful and can recognize other people's feelings. He can think abstractly, and it would not be difficult to have a conversation with him concerning such philosophical matters as death and the existence of God.

IX. Counseling Joe: A Developmental Perspective

If you were to counsel Joe, how might your knowledge of developmental theory affect your work with him?

X. Developing Your Own Developmental Theory

Based on each of the domains listed below, formulate your own developmental theory. Describe any common threads that exist among the development of the varying domains.

1. *Cognitive development:* Describe how you believe an individual develops his or her cognitive processes. Can you identify unique stages in which developmental milestones are reached? Do you think differences exist between the cognitive development of males and females?

2. *Physical development:* Describe the physical development of the individual. Can you identify unique stages in which developmental milestones are reached? Describe some of the differences you see of the physical development of males and females.

3. *Personality development:* Describe personality development. How does it take place? Can you identify unique stages in which developmental milestones are reached? Do you think differences exist between the personality development of males and females?

4. *Social development:* How do you believe one develops social awareness and social skills? Can you identify unique stages in which developmental milestones are reached? Do you think there are dramatic differences between the social development of males, females, and cultural groups? Explain.

5. *Spiritual development:* Describe one's spiritual development. Distinguish it from religious development. Can you identify unique stages in which developmental milestones are reached? Do you think differences exist between the spiritual development of males, females, and cultural groups? Explain.

XI. Examining Differing Perspectives on Abnormal Behavior

Respond to the following statements concerning abnormal behavior:
1. Make an argument for abnormal behavior being a function of early child-rearing. What early factors do you believe would affect later personality development?
2. Make an argument that the language used by families "creates" an environment for certain people to develop and exhibit maladaptive and abnormal behaviors. Describe how this happens
3. Using a genetic and biological orientation, make an argument for abnormal behavior being determined.

XII. Using the DSM
A. Reviewing Diagnostic Categories

Obtain a copy of DSM-IV-TR[2] (American Psychiatric Association, 2000). Pick one diagnostic category, and review the behavioral characteristics of that disorder. See if you can find some information on the etiology of that disorder. In class, discuss the varying diagnostic categories you found.

---

[2] If DSM-5 is published, try your best to respond to the questions based on the new manual.

B. Describing a Person Based on the Five Axes
1. The following describes a person using the five axes of the DSM-IV. Using the DSM, describe this person as best you can.

    Axis I: Adjustment Disorder with Depressed Mood (309.0)
    Axis II: Avoidant Personality Disorder (301.82)
    Axis III: Sickle-Cell Disease without Crisis (ICD-9-M: 282.61)
    Axis IV: Divorce
    Axis V: GAF = 60 (current); 75 (highest in past year)

2. In small groups, have each person develop their own five axes diagnosis. Then have the other group members describe the person.

C. Using the Five Axes of DSM-IV-TR
Examine the cases of Gloria (Box 9.3), Joe (Box 9.4), Kenny (Box 9.5), and Jason (Box 9.6) and describe each of them on the five axes of DSM-IV-TR.

Box 9.5: Kenny

Kenny is a 28-year-old male who was referred to this therapist due to feelings of depression as a result of the recent death of a friend from AIDS and the emergence of memories of being molested as a very young child by an adult male relative. In addition, he is currently questioning his sexual identity, which has been homosexual his whole adult life.

Kenny's mood has been depressed; however, despite a suicide attempt by ingestion of pills six months ago, he currently denies suicidal ideation and states he wants to "move on" with his life. Kenny has had a number of recent experiences, including seeing flashes of white light, black forms, feelings of something crawling on him, and feeling like he was "shocked." He believes that some of this may be related to feelings of guilt that are a result from his strict fundamentalist upbringing. He states that the guilt he has felt from his homosexual lifestyle may have caused him much stress, which manifested in some of the above symptoms. He describes his homosexual relationships as addictive and compulsive in nature. He has never had a long-term relationship.

Kenny is alert, oriented to time, place, and person, and verbal. He is quite open, easily sharing much about his life. His mood is moderately depressed, and he periodically sobs about the death of his friend, the guilt he feels about his homosexuality, and the memories of his sexual molestation. He seems coherent and his thinking seems clear. His conversations are clear and sharp. Although there are no clear indications of verbal or auditory hallucinations, seeing "white lights, black forms, and feelings things crawling on me" should be explored in more depth as possible hallucinatory material. It is unclear as to whether these are manifestations of a stressful period in his life, medical in nature, or possible hallucinations of a psychotic nature. He currently denies suicidal or homicidal ideation.

Box 9.6: Jason

Jason Reunter, thirteen, was brought in for counseling by his father due to feelings of depression and a drop in his grades within the last six months. He is the oldest of three children, having two younger sisters—Nicole, who is ten, and Stephanie, who is seven. Jason has been diagnosed as having Attention Deficit Disorder with Hyperactivity and Dyslexia. Until recently Jason obtained mostly A's and B's in school. Now, he is obtaining mostly C's in school. Over the years Jason has received assistance in a resource room for a math learning disability. Jason tends to be very well spoken, alert, and is described by teachers as "intellectually sharp." Jason has a fear of doctors and counselors, which his father relates back to Jason being treated for meningitis when he was four years old. The meningitis was successfully treated.

Jason's father, who is divorced, notes that he had always been satisfied in his marriage and was surprised when a couple of years ago his wife noted that she was unhappy. One year ago, he and his wife separated and they recently were divorced. Mr. Reunter believes his wife left him in order to "discover herself as she moved into a new stage in life" (he references Gail Sheehy's book, *Passages*). He notes that a year ago, his wife moved in with an "unemployed alcoholic," although she is currently not living with this man. Mr. Reunter has custody of the children, and he states that he is dealing with his own depression related to the loss of his marriage. Mr. Reunter works as a shoe salesman. He wonders if the recent divorce and his own feelings of depression are related to Jason's drop in grades and feelings of depression.

XIII. Classifying Medication in the Treatment of Emotional Problems
A. Identifying Psychotropic Medications

For each of the following categories, describe possible diagnostic classifications for which the drugs may be used. Then, give examples of some of the common medications in each of the categories.

1. <u>Antipsychotics</u>
   Description:

   Examples:

2. <u>Mood stabilizers</u>
   Description:

   Examples:

3. <u>Antidepressants</u>
   Description:

   Examples:

4. <u>Anti-anxiety</u>
   Description:

   Examples:

5. <u>Stimulants</u>
   Description:

   Examples:

B. Using Psychotropic Medications
Make an argument for and against the use of each of the broad categories of drugs listed in Exercise A. Discuss your answers in small groups in class.

XIV. Ethical, Legal, and Professional Vignettes
(The ACA's code is at www.counseling.org under "Resources"). In responding to the following, consider referring to the ACA's code.

1. A counselor discovers that a psychologist in his office is continually diagnosing individuals as having a serious pathology. The counselor, who believes that the psychologist is ignoring predictable developmental stressors, decides to complain to him about his procedures. Is the psychologist acting ethically? Professionally? Should the counselor complain? Should the counselor complain to an ethics board?
2. After discovering that an insurance company will not pay for a certain diagnosis, a licensed professional counselor decides to submit a similar, but not accurate, diagnosis in order to obtain insurance payments. If this is not done, the client will not be able to pay for her counseling sessions. Is this ethical? Professional? Legal?
3. A counselor believes the vast majority of individuals exhibiting signs of serious pathology can be treated in a proactive, humanistic manner, without medication. Is this ethical? Professional? Legal?
4. A graduate student in counseling who is hoping to become a school counselor complains to his professor that there is no reason to learn DSM-IV-TR (or DSM-5) or knowledge about psychopathology, for she is going to be working with relatively normal students and will not need to submit diagnoses to insurance companies. Is this rationale reasonable? Why or why not?
5. A counselor at a college counseling center insists on referring out all students who come to the center with symptoms that suggest serious pathology. Is this counselor acting wisely? Is this ethical? Professional?

6. A psychiatrist insists that *all* "patients" that have an Axis I or Axis II diagnosis on DSM-IV-TR (or DSM-5) (e.g., anything from a serious adjustment problem to severe psychopathology) should be on some form of medication. Is this position defendable? Is it ethical? Professional? Legal?
7. A counselor who is working with a moderately depressed client suggests that she needs to seriously consider taking anti-depressant medication. She then refers the client to a psychiatrist. Is this ethical? Professional? Legal?
8. An unlicensed counselor offers, for a fee, educational workshops to help individuals understand developmental tasks and unique developmental issues. Can the counselor ethically and legally do this?
9. A counselor places an ad in the local newspaper that states, "holistic, unintrusive, non-psychopathologically oriented counseling. See a counselor who cares and can offer hope to all individuals." Is this type of ad ethical? Professional? Legal?
10. A counselor who works with many special education students uses the DSM-IV-TR (or DSM-V) as an aid to parents in understanding their child's learning problems. Other counselors chastise this counselor and tell him that he is using a book that promotes psychopathology. Are these counselors on firm ground? Why or why not?
11. A counselor with whom you are acquainted tells you about a client of hers and describes her as having acute psychotic episodes. She describes her client as schizophrenic, and notes the following symptoms:

    The client says that she is possessed by a spirit, and has episodes of shouting, laughing, and weeping. In addition, she sometimes refuses to eat and will withdraw. Periodically, she says she even hits her head against a wall.

    After hearing this description, you realize that this client, who is from the Middle East, may be experiencing "Aara," a culture-bound syndrome that is not considered a sign of severe pathology in her country of origin. After explaining this to the counselor, she says to you, "Well, you can call this what you want, but the client is crazy." What should you do?
12. Despite the fact that some of your colleagues state that they want to work with clients from nondominant groups, you realize that these same colleagues have few clients of color on their caseloads; when they do see clients from nondominant groups, they seem to drop out of counseling more quickly than their other clients. What should you do?
13. A school counselor you know avoids working with students from nondominant groups, and when she does, she seems to be "stiff and nervous." You believe she is not conscious of her lack of comfort with diverse students. What should you do?
14. A counselor tells you that he is only going to work with clients from nondominant groups because he believes they are frequently misdiagnosed and are treated less competently by White counselors. He states that he will deny services to White clients. Is this ethical? Is this professional? Is this legal?

CHAPTER 10

CAREER DEVELOPMENT

I. Work, Avocations, Leisure Activities: What Are They?
A. Basic Definitions
Define the words *work*, *avocations*, and *leisure activities*. How are they the same? How are they different?

B. Satisfaction of Needs
In the space provided in Table 10.1, give examples of how work, avocations, and leisure may satisfy some of the needs listed.

Table 10.1: Needs Satisfied through Work, Avocations, and Leisure Activities

	Work	Avocation	Leisure Activities
Income			
Ego/Pride			
Self-Esteem			
Meaning			
Social			
Identity			

II. Very Early Memories: Connecting Early Interest to Career Interests Today
Think back to when you were about 6 years old and recall what you hoped to be when you "grew up." With your nondominant hand, draw a picture of yourself in that career. Again, with your nondominant hand and imagining you are 6, write a few sentences about what it would be like in that career. For example, someone might write, "I want to be a bus driver and drive all over the city," or "when I grow up, I am going to be a firefighter…" Next, again imagining you are 6, with your nondominant hand draw a picture of your parents and their work, and then write something about what they do. Share your picture and writing. What similarities and differences do you see in what you imagined you would be at 6 and your decision to go into counseling? In what ways did your parents' work and your early perceptions of their jobs influence your career dreams? How have those perceptions and your parents' influence changed for you through adolescence and your life to this point?

* This exercise was adapted from material by Dr. Cheree Hammond, Eastern Mennonite University. Her contribution is greatly appreciated.

III. Psychodynamic Factors and Career Choices

The kind of parenting you received undoubtedly affected your career choice. With this in mind, Box 10.1 examines the different parenting styles that Anne Roe believed were important in career choice. Examine these styles and identify one or two that most seem like the parenting you received. Reflect on whether or not that parenting style affected your occupational choice. Do the same exercise with one or two close friends or classmates.

Box 10.1: Parenting Styles and Occupational Choice

1. *Protective.* The parents are indulgent and demonstratively affectionate, and give the child special privileges. The home may be described as child centered. Children from such homes tend to gravitate to the service, arts, or entertainment fields.

2. *Demanding.* The parents set forth high expectations for accomplishment and impose strict regulation and obedience. Children growing up in this type of environment may be oriented to general culture (lawyers, teachers, scholars, librarians) or to the arts and entertainment fields.

3. *Rejecting.* The parents do not accept the child as a child, perhaps not even as an individual. They are often cold, hostile, and derogatory, making the child inferior and unaccepted. Rejected children tend to pursue science occupations.

4. *Neglecting.* The parents simply ignore the child; they give little attention, either positive or negative. They provide minimum physical care and less emotional sustenance. Neglected children tend to develop science and outdoor interests.

5. *Casual.* The parents give emotional and physical attention to the child, but only after higher-priority issues in their own lives have been attended to. Children treated casually tend to gravitate to technological occupations (engineers, aviators, applied scientists) or organizational occupations (bankers, accountants, clerks).

6. *Loving.* The parents are warm, helpful, and affectionate. They set limits and guide behavior through rational problem solving. They help the child with activities but are not intrusive. Children whose parents are loving tend to gravitate to service or business-contact occupations (promoters, salespeople). (Peterson, Sampson, & Reardon, 1991, pp. 55-56)

IV. Personality Development and Career Choices

Describe how each of the following has influenced your career choices:
1. Early child-rearing practices by your parents or guardians
2. Modeling by parents or guardians
3. Position in your family
4. Personality factors of siblings
5. Temperament (your biological tendencies toward certain personality traits)
6. Other early influences that may have affected your personality formation

V. Situational Factors and Career Choices

Describe how the following situational factors may have influenced your career choices:
1. Economic factors
2. Geographical factors
3. Health factors
4. Social and cultural factors
5. Other factors

VI. Developmental Tasks and Career Choices

A. Developmental Career Strategies

Your instructor will divide the class into small groups and assign each group to one of Super's (Super & Hall, 1978; Super, Savicaks, & Super, 1996) five developmental stages (growth, exploration, establishment, maintenance, and decline). On the basis of these stages, each group should devise strategies to assist individuals in their career development. (The same task can be completed for Super's substages.)

B. Assessing Your Developmental Stage

1. Box 10.2 is a checklist of the exploration stage of Super's developmental theory and was developed by Harris-Bowlsby, Spivack, and Lisansky (1991, p. 175). In this checklist, Super's exploration stage is broken down into crystallization, specification, and implementation tasks. Go through the checklist and identify those areas in which you have not completed a task leading to eventual career choice.

Box 10.2: Exploration Stage Checklist

	Not Yet Completed	Already Completed
Crystallization Tasks		
Realizing that I need to crystallize my alternative	☐	☐
Knowing how to organize occupations and programs of study in a meaningful way	☐	☐
Knowing what interests me	☐	☐
Knowing what my abilities/skills are	☐	☐
Knowing what my values are	☐	☐
Knowing how to use information about myself to focus my exploration of occupations and educational programs	☐	☐
Applying the steps of a planful decision-making process to my vocational and educational choices	☐	☐
Knowing which life roles I want to play	☐	☐
Identifying several occupations for detailed exploration	☐	☐
Identifying several educational programs for detailed exploration	☐	☐
Specification Tasks		
Selecting criteria that will assist in narrowing my occupational alternatives	☐	☐
Gathering detailed information about high-priority occupations and educational programs	☐	☐
Using information and criteria to make a tentative selection of occupational and educational programs	☐	☐
Declaring a major or choosing a program of study	☐	☐
Drafting plans to "reality test" three or more occupations	☐	☐
Implementation Tasks		
Drafting a plan for the implementation of possible educational or occupational choices	☐	☐
Learning and using job interviewing skills	☐	☐
Learning and using networking skills (to identify available jobs)	☐	☐
Finding a full-time job in the chosen occupation	☐	☐

If you believe you have successfully passed through the exploration stage, give this checklist to a client or friend for them to complete.

2. Greenhaus, Callanan, & Godhalk (2010) have taken Super's establishment stage and broken it down into what he calls early establishment, and achievement or late establishment. Box 10.3 is a checklist I have created based on these substages. Go through the checklist and identify those areas in which you have not completed a task leading to eventual career choice. If you believe you have successfully passed through the establishment stage, have a client or friend complete the checklist.

Box 10.3: Establishment Stage Checklist

	Not Yet Completed	Already Completed
Early Establishment Tasks		
I have settled fairly well into my career	☐	☐
I am beginning to feel settled in at work	☐	☐
I am beginning to feel a sense of belonging at work	☐	☐
I am just beginning to feel like I can periodically express controversial ideas at work	☐	☐
At my work setting, I am learning what I am good at	☐	☐
I am concerned with how well I will perform at work	☐	☐
To some degree, my sense of self is dependent on how I achieve at work	☐	☐
I often look to others for approval about how well I am doing at work	☐	☐
Achievement Tasks (Late Establishment Tasks)		
I am definitely "moving up" in my work setting	☐	☐
I am a creative and independent thinker at work	☐	☐
I add more than my share to the work environment	☐	☐
I feel good about who I am in my work setting	☐	☐
I am self-confident about my ability at work	☐	☐
I consciously attempt to take on positions of authority at work	☐	☐
I seek to satisfy myself, not others at work	☐	☐
I generally feel comfortable expressing my opinions at work	☐	☐

VII. What Planet Do You Come From?

An individual's personality is directly related to the kinds of interests that one holds and ultimately the kinds of choices one makes in career decision-making. Use the following exercise to determine your personality type. Imagine that you are on a spaceship traveling to another galaxy. When you get to this galaxy, you see three planets, each of which is occupied by two groups of people and each group has opposing qualities. Planet I is inhabited by individuals who are PAs or SLs, Planet II by EXs or INs, and Planet III by COs or ABs (see Box 10.4 for descriptions). As you go to each planet, which group of people do you gravitate toward?

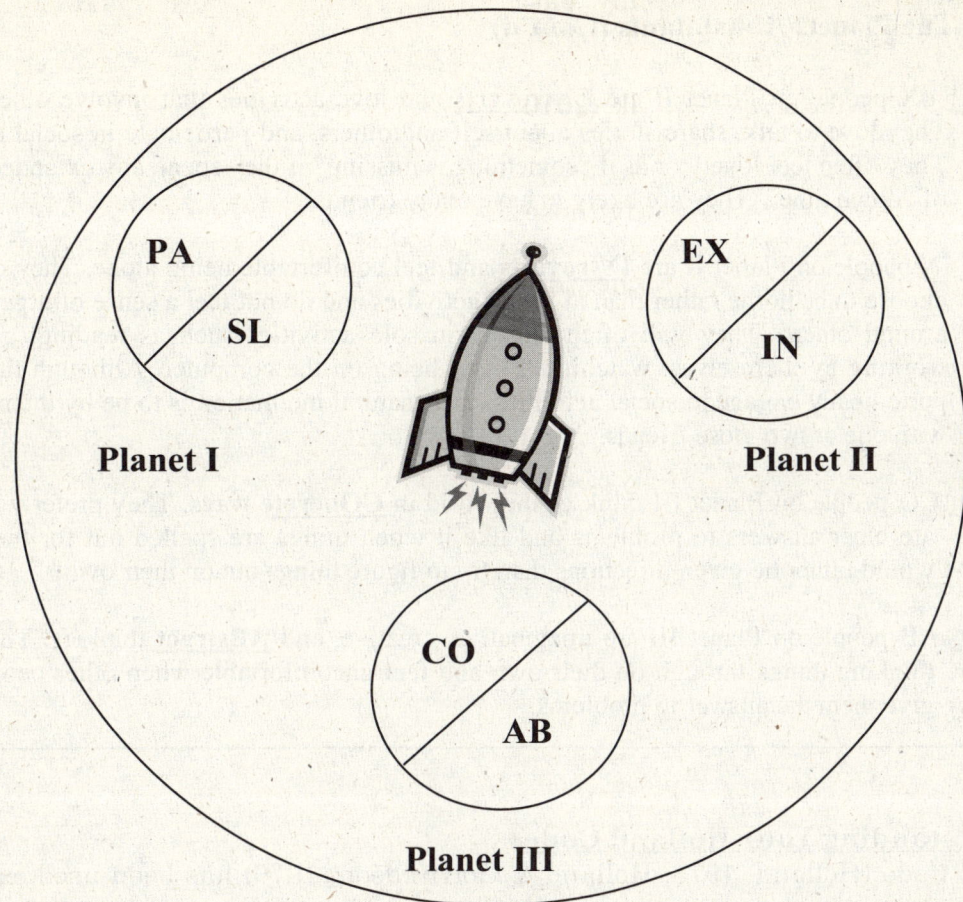

Assessment: After you have determined the three groups of people you tend to gravitate toward, rank order them. Then find other people in your class who have the same, or similar, rank order. Talk about your shared personality characteristics and then answer the questions listed below:

1. How do you think you came by your personality characteristics?
2. How do you think these characteristics have affected your career choices?
3. How do you think these characteristics will, in the future, affect your career choices?
4. How can knowledge of personality characteristics help you work with clients in their career decision-making process?

Box 10.4: The Planets' Inhabitants

<u>Planet PA:</u> PA people on Planet I love **Physical Activity**. Whenever they have an opportunity, they participate in some form of physical activity, including sports, hiking, yard work, exercise, or other related activities.

<u>Planet SL:</u> SL people on Planet I prefer a **Sedentary Lifestyle**. They'd rather participate in activities where they do not need to strain themselves. Although they might periodically like to go for a long work or work in the garden, they prefer doing such activities in slow and methodical ways.

> **Box 10.4: The Planets' Inhabitants (Cont'd)**
>
> **Planet EX:** EX people on Planet II are **EXtroverts** and love activities that involve other people. They love to talk, share stories about self and others, and participate in social activities. They often feel lonely or as if "something is missing" if they spend any extended amount of "down time." They are likely to have many friends.
>
> **Planet IN:** IN people on Planet II are **INtroverts** and feel comfortable being alone. They often will choose to be home rather than at social activities and do not feel a sense of urgency to be around others. They will often engage in solo activities such as reading, gardening, working by themselves, watching TV, or being on the computer. Although they might periodically engage in social activities, their natural inclination is to be by themselves or with one or two close friends.
>
> **Planet CO:** CO people on Planet III think of the world in **COncrete** ways. They prefer when there are clear answers to problems and like it when things are spelled out for them. They would rather be given directions than try to figure things out on their own.
>
> **Planet AB:** AB people on Planet III are imaginative, creative, and **ABstract** thinkers. They prefer thinking things through on their own and feel uncomfortable when other people try to give them the answer to problems.

VIII. Understanding Your Holland Code

The Holland Code (Holland, 1973; Holland & Gottfredson, 1976) has been used extensively to assist in matching one's personality type with occupations. Have your instructor help you determine a Holland Code by administering one of the established interest inventories, such as the "self-directed search" or the "strong interest inventory." After you have determined your code, read the section entitled "Understanding Your Code" in Appendix G. Then, find students with similar codes and discuss the following:

1. What personality factors do you share in common?
2. What similar occupational interests do you share?*
3. How does knowledge of your code confirm or question your decision to be a counselor?
4. How could you use the Holland Code when working with clients?

* You may want to use the *Dictionary of Holland Occupational Codes* (Gottfredson, Holland, & Ogawa, 1996) to assist you in examining occupations you might find interesting. Or, do an Internet search of Holland Code jobs.

IX. Social-Cognitive Career Theory (SCCT)

Anchored in self-efficacy theory, SCCT states that the types of choices we make are based on our current beliefs about whether we can perform certain behaviors (Lent, 2005; Patton & McIlveen, 2009). SCCT suggests that self-efficacy is related to our family experiences (e.g., what we're told we're good at), sociological influences (e.g., discrimination, mobility, sexism, and the economy), our abilities and aptitudes, our interests, our sense of our personality style (e.g., the kinds of work environments we most comfortably seem to fit in), and the goals we have in life. SCCT also suggests that individuals are affected by objective factors and perceived environmental factors For instance, economic hardship, educational experiences, and societal factors (e.g., societal values around gender, culture, disability status, etc.) are objective factors that all affect the kinds of choices available to a person. However, such factors are also affected by one's unique cognitive filters (e.g., a person with a disability is affected by discrimination, but is also affected by his or her perception of self and of discrimination). Given the above, respond to the following:

1. How have beliefs about your career path been shaped by parents, family, culture, and society?
2. How have your beliefs about your career path been shaped by your abilities and aptitudes?
3. How have your beliefs about your career been shaped by your interests and personality?
4. Do you think the above beliefs are intractable; that is, do they represent who you are and you cannot change them? Or, do you believe that you may be able to, and even want to, change some of your beliefs about self?
5. If you were to change some of the beliefs about yourself, which would they be? How might changing your beliefs affect your career decisions?

X. Constructivist Career Development

Constructivist career development is a post-modern approach to career counseling that questions an individual's "truth" about self relative to his or her career development (Gysbers et al., 2009; Hutchison & Niles, 2009; Schultheiss, 2007). Constructivists believe that through conversations with career counselors, individuals can begin to understand the dominant narratives (life stories) that drive their lives and push them to certain career decisions. Dominant narratives that are detrimental to a person can be deconstructed and new narratives can be constructed. Counselors can work to understand each person's unique narratives, help them construct new narratives, and also work on changing dominant societal language and the resulting barriers they create that differentially affect minorities and women. With this in mind, respond to the following:

1. What narratives dominate your life relative to the career choices you have made?

2. Are any of these narratives detrimental to the kinds of choices you have made or will make?

3. Are there ways for you to deconstruct or limit your dominant, detrimental narratives?

4. Are there new narratives that you can develop? Are there individuals who can help you do this?

XI. Integrating Career Development Theories

Read the story of Roger in Box 10.6 and then answer the following questions that address many of the theories of career development discussed in this chapter:

1. What early parenting styles affected Roger's career choices?
2. What family factors affected Roger's career choices?
3. How have situational factors affected Roger's career choices?
4. How does "fit" in a job play a role in Roger's life?
5. What developmental tasks affected Roger's career choices?
6. How has Roger's beliefs about his abilities affected the choices he has made?
7. Do you believe that Roger's beliefs are based on fact or on self-perception?

> **Box 10.6: Roger**
>
> Roger states that he always knew he would go to college and obtain a graduate degree. Being the oldest of five children, he was often given responsibility for taking care of his younger siblings and was seen as the child who would "make it big" in life.
>
> For many years, Roger was convinced he wanted to work in some aspect of religion. This was reinforced by his "strict religious upbringing," which included very religious parents, friends who all shared the same religion, and a commitment to a fundamentalist church that also reinforced his beliefs. Roger felt as if he was good interpersonally and believed he had a calling to preach to others. He also "knew" he had the path to truth and happiness and wanted to tell others about this path. However, when Roger started college, he found that his beliefs were challenged. He suddenly had an identity crisis as he pondered what else he could do. Having grown up on a farm and worked with animals, for a short time, he considered becoming a veterinarian. However, he decided not to pursue this interest because he believed his grades were not good enough to get into veterinary school, and he knew he would have to transfer schools and be away from his girlfriend. Therefore, having always done well in math and believing he had good interpersonal skills, he decided to major in math education and joined ROTC for the financial aid afforded through the GI bill.
>
> Although Roger wanted to enter pilot training, he was told that he would have to commit to the Air Force for five years, a commitment he did not wish to make. So, he took a job in meteorology, which required only a three-year commitment. Roger so enjoyed meteorology that he began to consider a career in the Air Force as a meteorologist. He became enthused about the field, received his master's degree, and traveled the world. Continually promoted, Roger practiced meteorology in the Air Force for 18 years.
>
> Wanting a change, Roger then took a job as head of ROTC at a large Midwestern university and later worked at officer assignment in personnel. Then, after 24 years in the Air Force and having seen some friends become bitter and others start drinking too much, Roger began to feel that the Air Force was "not fun anymore." He retired from the Air Force, and pursued a master's degree in business administration (M.B.A.). He subsequently took a position at the financial aid office at the university where he now works.
>
> Feeling like he couldn't relate to others in the financial aid office and increasingly feeling a sense of disenchantment with his M.B.A., Roger decided to quit his master's degree and took a job in freshman advising. Finding he really enjoyed academic advising and wanting skills to match what he was doing, he started his master's degree in counseling. He is now considering obtaining a job as a school counselor. However, he is afraid he will not be able to find a job due to his age.

8. What narratives have driven Roger's life?
9. Are there any narratives that might have been detrimental to Roger's career choices?
10. What societal prejudices may have affected the choices Roger has made or will make?
11. What role do you believe counselors play in advocating for the elimination of societal prejudices that can affect a client's career choices?
12. If you were to work with Roger, what might be most beneficial for him?

XII. Understanding the Career Development of Others

In an effort to understand the career development process, ask an individual in an occupation of your choice the following questions:

1. How long have you held this job?
2. Do you view your current job as part of your career or as a transitory job?
3. If you view this job as part of your career, when did you first think about doing it?
4. What aspects of your occupation motivate you to stay in it or leave it (e.g., money, support, etc.)?
5. What early family factors affected your eventual career choices?
6. What personality factors do you believe you hold that make you particularly suited or not suited for this occupation?
7. What situational factors affected your career choices?
8. What interests, abilities, and values do you hold that make you particularly suited for this job?
9. Looking back on your life, do you think that you might have "bought into" some beliefs about yourself that were not true but were espoused by family, friends, and society (e.g., women are told they are not good at math although they have the aptitude)?
10. After reflecting on the last question (item 9), what beliefs and narratives about yourself affected your eventual decision to pursue this occupation and to not pursue other occupations?

XIII. Exploring Occupational Information

A. O*NET, DOT, and OOH

Choose three occupations and use O*NET, the *Dictionary of Occupational Titles* (DOT), and the *Occupational Outlook Handbook* (OOH), to discover details about them. In small groups discuss the kind of information available at each of these sites as well as some of the more interesting facts about the occupations you researched. Use the following websites in finding your information:

1. DOT: http://www.occupationalinfo.org/
2. O*NET: http://online.onetcenter.org/
3. OOH: http://www.bls.gov/oco/

B. University Career Counseling Centers

Visit the Career Counseling Center at your college or university and do the following:

1. Take a computerized career assessment instrument and describe its strengths and weaknesses in class.
2. Examine other occupational information at the center.
3. Find out what other services the Career Counseling Center offers.

C. Career Counselors in Private Practice

Visit a private practice career counselor, find the answers to the following questions, and discuss what you found in class:

1. What services does this counselor offer?
2. What degrees and credentials does he or she have?
3. What kinds of assessment instruments are available from this counselor?
4. What kinds of occupational information are available?
5. What theories of career counseling does this person adhere to?

D. Elementary, Middle, or High School Counselor
Visit an elementary, middle, or secondary school counselor, find the answers to the following questions, and discuss what you found in class:
1. What kinds of career services does this counselor offer?
2. How are the services based on a developmental model of career counseling?
3. What kinds of assessment instruments are available from this counselor?
4. What kinds of occupational information are available for the students?
5. What theories of career counseling does this person adhere to?

XIV. Assisting a Client (or Yourself) in Understanding Career Choices
A. Identifying Potential Jobs
Have a client (or you) do one or more of the following activities to explore job options:
1. Complete select exercises from among Exercises I–XIII in this chapter.
2. Take an interest inventory and have it interpreted.
3. Look through the newspaper want ads and write down all jobs that seem interesting.
4. Based on the knowledge you learned about yourself, use the DOT, O*NET, or OOH and develop an expanded list (perhaps 20 to 50 jobs) of potential occupations (see Exercise XIII for websites).
5. From the knowledge gained from doing items 1 through 4, rank order the top 5 or 10 jobs. Starting with the one that is ranked highest and go on informational interviews with as many as those occupations that may seem like potential career choices.

B. Identifying Skills Needed for Your List of Occupations
From the list in Exercise A, starting with the top-ranked occupation, have your client (or you) write down the jobs on the left side of the page of Table 10.2, and identify the skills needed for those jobs in the space provided (use the *DOT*, *O*NET,* and *OOH* if you need help identifying skills). Then decide if your client (or you) currently has the skills needed for the job and, if not, what can be done to obtain the skills. See the example in Table 10.2.

XV. Ethical, Legal, and Professional Vignettes
(The ACA's code is at www.counseling.org under "Resources"). In responding to the following, consider referring to the ACA's code.

1. It is not unusual for individuals who have little or no training in career development to be offering workshops on career issues, testing for career decision-making, and even career counseling. What do you think of this practice? Is it ethical? Professional? Legal?
2. A master's level social worker you know tells you that he is doing career counseling with some of his clients. You know that social workers rarely, if ever, get specific training in career counseling. What should you do? Is this ethical? Professional? Legal?

Table 10.2: Occupational Skills Identification

Job	Needed Skills	Have Skills?	How to Get Skills
Counselor	Interviewing	Yes	Practice sessions, role-play
	Empathy	Partly	Take courses, get info from agencies
	Record keeping	No	Take courses, reflect, read books/journals
	Theory knowledge	Partly	Role-play, internship, take skills classes
	Counseling	Partly	Take course/internship
	Consulting	No	Take course/internship, speak to consultants about their jobs
	Testing	No	Take course, take tests, practice
	Research	No	Take course, read journals, join organizations, do research
	Group skills	No	Take courses, practicum, internship, participate in group

3. A counselor working with an African-American client on career development issues tells you that she thinks the client is making excuses for not finding a job. The client, she says, insists that there is little upward mobility for a "lower-class, undereducated, Black person." Is there any truth to what the client says? Would you say anything to this counselor? Is she acting ethically? Professionally?

4. An elementary counselor you know continues to use gender-specific language when referring to certain occupations (e.g., fireman rather than firefighter). In addition, he tends to push girls toward traditionally female occupations and boys toward traditionally male occupations. You mention that you think he might want to change his language and ways of acting with the students, and he says, "This is how the world is. Why should I give them a false image?" What should you do? Is he acting ethically? Professionally?

5. A middle-school counselor you know insists on having students make career decisions despite the fact that developmentally, they should be exploring their strengths and weaknesses and examining the different kinds of occupations in the world of work. How should you approach this situation? Is the counselor acting ethically? Professionally?
6. A high school counselor you know spends considerable time assisting high-achieving students with college-bound issues. He spends little time working on career and vocational counseling for other students. What should you do? Is this ethical? Professional?
7. A counselor in private practice is working with a client who was recently laid off from her job. The counselor has given the client a diagnosis of "adjustment reaction with anxiety features." This diagnosis assures payment by the client's insurance company. The sole focus of counseling is career issues. Is this ethical? Professional? Legal?
8. A colleague of yours insists on using a psychodynamic approach to career counseling that has not been shown to be effective. As a psychodynamic therapist, he insists that you can't "measure unconscious motivation." Is he acting ethically? Professionally?
9. You work at the Career Management Center at your university, and the director has insisted that no counselors should be spending more than two half-hour sessions with clients. She says that all of the information these days for finding jobs is on computers, and counselors should simply help students learn how to use the computer. You believe that career counseling is an intensive career development process. What should you do?
10. The Community Mental Health Center where you work insists on down-playing career issues and playing up "intrapsychic and systemic" issues. You tell your supervisor that you believe the world of work is crucial to the development of a positive self-concept. The supervisor tells you that if you believe that way, you might want to consider finding a job someplace else. Has the supervisor acted ethically? Professionally? Legally? What should you do?
11. A colleague of yours is a "feminist career counselor" and as such, often tells her female clients that they have been hoodwinked into believing that they could not be successful at traditional male occupations, such as construction worker, physician, mathematician, and so on. Do you believe that what she is doing is ethical? Professional? Does she have a point?
12. An elementary school counselor continues to coordinate career day for her school and bring in "traditional" careers, such as firefighter, police officer, lawyer, and doctor. What are your thoughts about the counselor expanding these choices? What are the positives and drawbacks to offering a much broader view of occupational choice?

CHAPTER 11

RESEARCH AND EVALUATION

I. Understanding Paradigm Shifts
Kuhn's (1962) concept of the paradigm shift states that knowledge builds upon itself and that new discoveries are based on the evolution of past knowledge. When current knowledge does not adequately explain the way things work, then the time is ripe for a change in our understanding of the world—ripe for a paradigm shift. Without research, knowledge remains stagnant, and new paradigms are unlikely to evolve. The following exercise challenges our traditional way of viewing the world and is a metaphor for the importance of making paradigm shifts. Your task is to connect the nine dots with four straight lines without lifting the pen or pencil from the paper (see solution at end of chapter).*

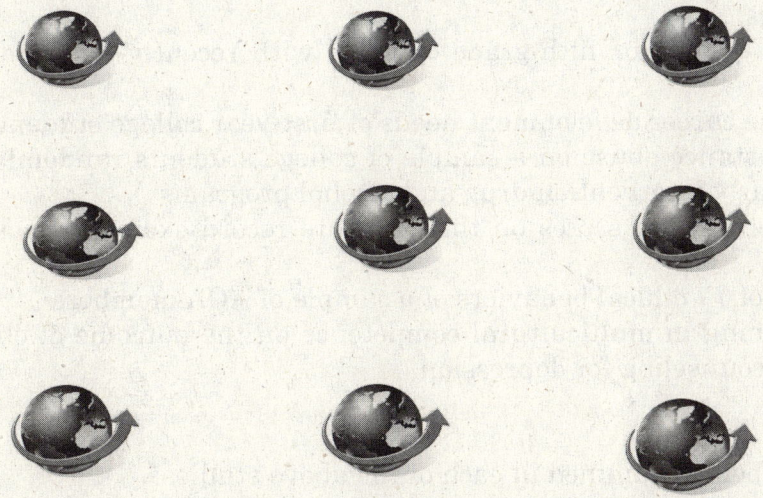

* This exercise is compliments of Dr. Paddy Kennington, LPC, NCC, certified EMDR therapist. Her contribution is greatly appreciated. Exercise found in Watzwalick, Weakland, & Fisch (1974).

II. Conducting a Literature Search
Pick a topic of your choice and conduct an electronic search using a database such as ERIC, PsychINFO, etc. Gather your information, and write a two- to four-page, double-spaced literature review. Share your literature review in class.

III. Identifying Variables of Quantitative Research Studies
A. Variables
Using the short descriptions listed below, identify the variables of the studies. In your answer, determine whether the study has one or more independent variables, dependent variables (outcome variable), variables that are related to one another but are not clearly an independent or dependent variable, or a descriptive variable that can be analyzed through survey research:

1. The effect of aerobic exercise on depression of individuals in a beginning aerobics class
2. The effect of two types of aerobic exercise classes on depression and anxiety of individuals in a beginning aerobics class
3. The effect of two types of aerobic classes and three forms of music on anxiety and depression of individuals in an advanced aerobics class
4. The relationship between empathy and unconditional positive regard of beginning counseling students
5. The relationship between multicultural counselor training and sensitivity toward clients of different cultures
6. An examination of the types of ethical complaints made against licensed professional counselors
7. An examination of the frequency of counselors' attendance in their own therapy
8. The effect of anti-depressant medication on depression
9. The effect of counseling and the use of anti-depressant medication on depression
10. A survey of the theoretical orientation of school counselors, agency counselors, and college counselors
11. The impact of a "group for fifth-grade children with recently divorced parents" on their self-esteem
12. An analysis of the career development needs of first-year college students
13. The effect of substance abuse on a sample of college students randomly assigned to three different early intervention drug and alcohol programs
14. The relationship between scores on the graduate record exam and achievement in graduate school
15. The perceptions of 77 ethical behaviors of a sample of ACA members
16. The effect of raining in multicultural competence on the outcome of clients of color who are in brief counseling for depression

B. Population
Identify the population being examined in each of the above studies.

IV. Developing Hypotheses and Research Questions
Using the descriptions in Exercise III, develop a research question, a null hypothesis, and/or a directional hypothesis for each study listed.

V. Steps You Might Use in Developing a Qualitative Study
Describe some of the steps and tools you might use to conduct the following four types of qualitative studies.

A. Grounded Theory (some possible tools: focus groups, observation, questions, coding, note-taking, purposeful samples, coding)
1. The development of a theoretical orientation in counselors
2. The definition of empathic responding by physicians
3. Defining multicultural competence in counselors

B. Phenomenological Designs (some possible tools: focus groups, questions, examination of "stories," coding, note-taking, purposeful samples)
1. Understanding posttraumatic disorders of survivors of Hurricane Katrina
2. Common elements among survivors of childhood molestation
3. Experiences of first generation Latino/Latina clients in counseling

C. Ethnographic Studies (some possible tools: participant observation, interviews, document and artifact collection)
1. The kinds of facilitative behaviors shown toward others by counselors at counselor conferences
2. Nonverbal behavior of Native Americans
3. The social behaviors of children with intellectual disabilities

D. Historical Research (some possible tools: literature reviews; oral histories; documents such as diaries, autobiographies, journals and magazines; films, recordings, paintings, and institutional records such as books, maps, buildings, artifacts)
1. The development of empathy as a counseling tool by helping professionals
2. The formation of the counseling profession
3. The use of symbols in healing

VI. Critiquing a Journal Article
Critique an article from a counseling journal using the following criteria:
1. Was this a quantitative or qualitative study?
2. What kind of quantitative or qualitative study was this? Be specific.
3. What made this the kind of study you stated it was in question 2?
4. Was there an adequate review of literature?
5. Was the hypothesis or research question firmly based on the literature review?
6. What results were found?
7. How was the study analyzed (e.g., types of statistics used)?
8. What are the implications of the results?
9. What future research might arise out of this research?
10. Generally, what did you think of the article?

VII. Designing a Research Study
Your instructor will divide the class into groups of three to five students. Choosing one of the research designs listed below, or another design discussed in class, have each group design a research study concerning the effectiveness or impact of counselors with their clients. Make sure that each group addresses, (1) how it would complete its literature review; (2) the design of the study; (3) the methodology of the study (participants, the exact steps of the study, the instruments or tools you would use to complete your study); and (4) the kind of statistical analysis that might be used in your study.

A. Quantitative Research: Experimental Designs
1. True experimental
2. Quasi-experimental research
3. One-shot case study and one group pretest/post-test design

B. Quantitative Research: Non-Experimental Designs
1. Correlational
2. Survey
3. *Ex post facto* (causal-comparative)

C. Qualitative Research
1. Grounded theory research
2. Phenomenological research
3. Ethnographic research
4. Historical research

VIII. Validating Qualitative Research

The ability to show trustworthy and credible results in qualitative research is based on how well the researcher is able to accurately record information and analyze results. The following suggests some ways to assure the credibility of the qualitative research (Best & Kahn, 2006; Christensen & Brumfield, 2010; McMillan & Schumacher, 2010). Your instructor will assign you an article based one of the following forms of qualitative research: grounded theory research, phenomenological research, ethnographic research, and historical research. Then, using the questions below, assess its quality:

1. If field works was involved, was it prolonged and persistent?
2. Was *triangulation*, or multiple methods, used in obtaining information (e.g., observation, interviewing, document collection)?
3. If participants were interviewed, was language used that the participants could understand?
4. Was information obtained described in clear and concrete terms?
5. Were multiple perspectives actively sought?
6. Were multiple researchers used to lessen bias?
7. Was there an attempt to "bracket off" one's own biases so such biases would not interfere with data gathering?
8. Were interviews mechanically recorded to assure accuracy?
9. Was an "informant" (a participant checker) or a researcher who was a participant observer used to corroborate evidence obtained?
10. Was an "outside auditor" used to check for biases in the research process
11. Were *member checks* that asked individuals who were interviewed to review transcripts for accuracy used?
12. Did the researchers actively look for discrepant data or information that did not support a particular point of view (such information offers a differing view of the "truth" of the situation)?
13. Were primary sources used as much as reasonable and possible?
14. Was there a rigorous process of reviewing the data, synthesizing results, and drawing conclusions and generalizations?

IX. Threats to Internal Validity in Quantitative Research

In conducting all types of experimental research, there are many threats to internal validity that can result in researchers coming to false conclusions about their study, if certain factors are not controlled (see Campbell & Stanley, 1963; Cook & Campbell, 1979; Shadish, Cook, & Campbell, 2002). Take each of the threats to internal validity listed in Box 11.1, and describe how a study might not control for it.

> **Box 11.1: Threats to Internal Validity**
>
> 1. *Ambiguous temporal precedence*, in which it is not clear which variable came first, thus yielding confusion about which was the cause and which was the effect.
> 2. *Selection*, in which the ways that subjects are selected and assigned to treatment groups causes differences in those groups, thus clouding whether differences found are the result of the treatment or of selection.
> 3. *History*, in which external events occur during the research that affects the treatment and results in invalid conclusions.
> 4. *Maturation*, in which maturational changes in subjects, such as growing older or more tired or becoming hungry, affect the results.
> 5. *Regression*, where there is a statistical tendency for extreme scores to move closer to the mean if tested a second time. Therefore, regardless of the effect of the treatment, treatment groups with particularly high or low pretest scores may have scores move toward the mean during post-testing, thus leading to false readings concerning the effect of the treatment.
> 6. *Attrition*, as when participants differentially drop out of treatment, thus leaving only the "better" or "worse" participants and results that are falsely attributed to the treatment.
> 7. *Testing*, in which exposure to a test can affect the results, such as when a knowledge of the pretest affects the results of the post-testing.
> 8. *Instrumentation*, where changes in the instrument(s) can affect the results, such as when a more difficult pretest is used, thus leading to the false conclusion that there were gains in post-testing.
> 9. *Additive and interactive effects of threats to internal validity*, when two or more threats to internal validity operate simultaneously and their joint or combined threat affects the results differently or more powerfully than either threat on its own.

X. Designing a Qualitative Study

Using the description below, answer the questions that follow concerning the development of a qualitative study on female genital mutilation in the United States:

> In recent years, there has been an uproar in many countries concerning the act of female genital mutilation (FGM), which occurs mostly in some parts of Africa, the Middle East, and Far East (Religious Tolerance, 2008). The practice generally includes anything from a partial clitoridectomy to excision of the clitoris, the inner labia, and the skin of the outer labia. In some cases, the remaining skin is stitched, leaving a tiny opening that makes it difficult to urinate, leaves the women prone to infections, and acts as a kind of chastity belt (World Health Organization, 2010). The procedure, which typically occurs at around age 7, symbolizes the induction into adulthood, reduces or eliminates sexual pleasure, and often results in painful sexual intercourse. Despite laws against such FGM in the United States, in some cases, it is still practiced.

1. What type of qualitative study would you design (grounded theory research, phenomenological research, ethnographic research, or historical research)?
2. Explain the steps you would use in actually doing your study.
3. How would you "bracket off" your own beliefs about this procedure in order to not have your biases interfere with your results?
4. In addition to bracketing off your own beliefs, what other ways might you use to assure limit biases in your results?

5. How would you gather your results?
6. What ethical and legal implications would you have to deal with?

XI. Designing a Quantitative Study

Using the description below, answer the questions that follow concerning the development of a quantitative study on counselors perceptions of ethical behaviors:

> What is ethical counselor behavior one year, may not be ethical the next. For instance, the most recent ethics code of the American Counseling Association (ACA, 2005) demonstrates how a code can change by including a number of revisions that challenge counselors to work in new ways. For instance, the code replaces the term "serious and foreseeable harm" with "clear and eminent danger," increases the restrictions on romantic and sexual relationships, softens the admissibility of dual relationships, includes a statement on end-of-life care for terminally ill clients, increases attention to social and cultural issues, allows counselors to refrain from making a diagnosis, highlights the importance of having a scientific basis for treatment modalities, requires counselors to have a transfer plan for clients, adds guidelines for how and when to use technology, and includes a statement about the right to confidentiality for deceased clients (ACA, 2005; Kaplan, et al., 2009).

1. What type of quantitative study might you design to examine counselors' perceptions of or reactions to ethical behaviors?
2. Explain the steps you would use in actually doing your study.
3. Explain how you would control for internal validity (see Box 11.1).
4. How would you gather your results?
5. How would you explain you're lack of control of some aspects of internal validity in your discussion section?
6. What ethical and legal implications would you have to deal with?

XII. Comparing Quantitative and Qualitative Research

In the space provided in Table 11.1, write how quantitative and qualitative research addresses the item in the first column.

XIII. Evaluating an Evaluation Form

A. University Evaluation Form

Most colleges and universities have some form of course evaluation that is completed at the end of the semester. Obtain a copy of the evaluation form used at your college and discuss any positive and negative aspects of that form.

B. Agency Evaluation Form

Visit a local social service agency and see whether the agency has any evaluation forms that are used to assess client satisfaction, the effectiveness of programs, and/or the overall effectiveness of the agency. Share these forms in class.

Table 11.1: Distinctions between Quantitative and Qualitative Research

	Quantitative	Qualitative
Assumptions About the World		
How Knowledge Is Applied		
Research Methods Used		
Biases and Validity		
Goals and Generalizability		
Researcher Role		
End Product		

XIV. Developing an Evaluation Form
A. Formative Evaluation (Process Evaluation)
In small groups or as a class, develop a formative (process) evaluation tool for your class.

B. Summative Evaluation (Outcome Evaluation)
In small groups or as a class, develop a summative (outcome) evaluation tool for your class.

XV. Writing a Fictitious Manuscript Describing a Research Study or Program Evaluation
In small groups, using APA style manual (6th ed.), write a fictitious manuscript or program evaluation as if you were submitting the manuscript to a journal for publication. Include the headings listed below. The manuscript should be based on a quantitative or qualitative research design or a program evaluation. Use the guidelines that follow:
1. *Title page:* Write a title page using APA style.
2. *Abstract:* Write an abstract that is no greater than 120 words.
3. *Introduction:* Use the same title that is listed on your title page, and then write the introductory section of the manuscript as if you had conducted a literature review. Make up your citations and include them in the literature review and place them in your reference list. Refer to your *APA Style Manual* for accurate display of citations.
4. *Method:* Include sections entitled "Participants," "Materials," and "Procedure." Make up the actual methods section.

5. *Results:* Make up your results.
6. *Discussion:* Write a discussion section as if you had actually completed the study.
7. *References:* Referring to your APA style manual and using your citations, make up a variety of references (e.g., books, articles, online, etc.).

XVI. Comparing Different Kinds of Research and Evaluation

Using the grid in Table 11.2, compare and contrast the different kinds of research and evaluation listed.

XVII. Ethical, Legal, and Professional Vignettes

(The ACA's code is at www.counseling.org under "Resources"). In responding to the following, consider referring to the ACA's code.

1. Recently, there has been research on the effectiveness of various drugs to combat the Human Immunodeficiency Virus (HIV). To test effectiveness, a drug company obtains permission to randomly assign individuals who have tested HIV-positive to two groups. One group will obtain a new drug, and the second group will obtain the existing drugs. Individuals do not know to which group they belong. Is this ethical? Professional? Legal?
2. What if the new drug treatment in vignette 1 shows promise for the treatment of HIV and AIDS? Do the researchers have a responsibility to stop the study and treat the control group, or should they allow the control group to finish its trials? Why or why not?
3. Based on the available research, a counselor, who works at a 30-day rehabilitation center for chemically dependent individuals starts a program that uses confrontation and humiliation. Although individuals can theoretically leave at any time, in this program, those who do not admit to their addictions and who do not begin to make major changes in their lives are heavily confronted by the whole group, are forced to shave their heads, and during "social time," are made to sit in their rooms and think about their lives. Is this ethical? Professional? Legal?
4. To become more familiar with a local community religious group, a counselor decides to become a participant observer and spends a week with the community at their retreat center. Part of their ritual is to ingest hallucinogenic mushrooms and to smoke marijuana during meditation times. Following the week at the center, he reports his experience to his supervisor, who reports the group to the local law enforcement agency for the illegal use of drugs. Is this ethical? Professional? Legal?
5. A counselor receives negative feedback via formative and summative evaluations about a workshop she presented to lower socioeconomic parents that focused on communicating with their teenagers. After reading the evaluations, the counselor decides, "They really didn't want to learn how to communicate with their kids. I simply won't do workshops on this topic for 'those people' any more. Next time, I'll present it to middle-class parents." Is this ethical? Legal? Professional?
6. A colleague of yours is working on her doctorate and has decided to do a pilot study that involves asking graduate students in counseling to take an interest inventory that measures one's personality orientation toward the world of work as well as a test that measures introversion/extroversion. She is hoping to show a relationship between the two scales. Your colleague forgoes asking permission of the human subjects committee of the university because she believes the study does not present a danger to the students. Is she acting ethically? Professionally? Legally?

Table 11.2: Comparing Different Kinds of Research and Evaluation

	Quantitative					Qualitative				Evaluation	
	Experimental:	Non-Experimental									
	True, Quasi, One-Shot/One Group Pre-Post	Correlational: Biovariate (Simple/Predictive) Multivariate	Survey	Ex Post Facto (Causal-Comparative)	Grounded Theory	Phenomeno-logical	Ethnographic	Historical	Formative (Process)	Summative (Outcome)
Focus										
Purpose										
Hypotheses/ Questions										
Population										
Design/Statistics										
Validity/ Credibility/ Trustworthiness										

7. In conducting research on fear response, one group of college students is told to place a hand in a box where they will touch a "friendly" animal, a second group is told to place a hand in the box and asked to "tell me what you feel," while a third group is told to place their hands in the box and asked to "tell me what the snake in the box feels like." All groups feel the same garden snake in the box. During the experiment, many of the students experience fear and have serious panic reactions. After the study, all students are "debriefed" to assure that they are feeling okay. Is this study ethical? Is it legal? Does it involve deception? When can a study ethically use deception?

8. In conducting a study to examine the effects of counselor response to clients from nondominant groups, the researcher only includes White males as counselors. Is this ethical? Professional? Legal?

9. In conducting the study in vignette 8, the researcher only includes African Americans as the "minority" clients. Is this ethical? Professional? Legal?

10. While conducting research on multiculturalism in counseling, a researcher bases his hypothesis on select research and ignores other research that would not support the hypothesis. The researcher states that this is ethical as there is enough research in the literature to support his point of view. Is this ethical? Professional? Legal?

11. A researcher conducts a "mixed methods," quantitative and qualitative analysis that examines the efficacy of immersion techniques in a multicultural counseling course. The quantitative analysis shows that the students become more sensitive to multicultural issues after immersion techniques, and the qualitative results show that the students deal with an extreme amount of anxiety in anticipation of doing the immersion activity. How might the two results complement one another? Are there any ethical considerations that one should consider based on these results?

12. A counselor who has obtained a national reputation for offering workshops on parenting skills does not provide a method for the workshop participants to evaluate her. She justifies this by saying, "I've done this a thousand times, and everyone always enjoys it." Does she have a point? Is this ethical? Professional?

13. Consistently receiving mediocre ratings when teaching a course on research, a counselor educator states, "Students never like research. I don't expect to get high ratings." Does he have a point? Is this ethical? Professional?

14. You have noticed that students in your classes tend to evaluate their professors based on how much they like them, not how much they learn. Should you do anything? Is this ethical? Professional?

Answer to Exercise I:

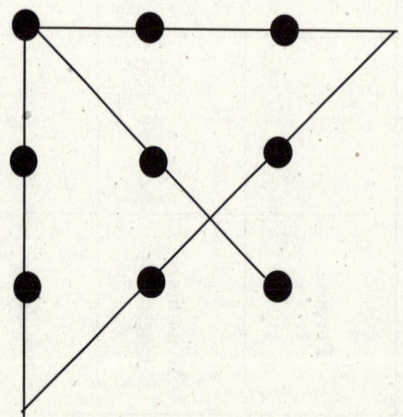

CHAPTER 12

TESTING AND ASSESSMENT

I. Differences between Testing and Assessment
In small groups or as a class, discuss the difference between testing and assessment. Give examples of some tests and of some assessment procedures.

II. Sharing Experiences with Testing
In class, discuss any positive or negative experiences you have had relative to taking a test.

III. Advantages and Disadvantages to Testing and Assessment
In small groups, discuss the items listed below. Then, pick a spokesperson and report back to the class. Your instructor will write on the board the advantages and disadvantages that are noted by the groups.
1. The advantages and disadvantages of cognitive ability tests like the SATs and GREs
2. The advantages and disadvantages of group achievement tests
3. The advantages and disadvantages of individual intelligence testing
4. The advantages and disadvantages of personality assessment
5. The advantages and disadvantages of diagnosis using the DSM-IV-TR (or DSM-5)

IV. Types of Tests
A. Identifying Types of Tests
Tests can either be criterion-referenced or norm-referenced and standardized or non-standardized. In small groups or as a class, place the name of the type of test category in the appropriate space.

1. _____ are those instruments in which the individual can compare his or her score to the conglomerate scores of a peer group.
2. _____ tests are designed to assess specific learning goals of an individual. Such tests show mastery of the subject matter at hand.
3. _____ are those assessment instruments that are administered in the same manner and under the same conditions each time they are given.
4. _____ procedures are not necessarily given under the same conditions and in the same manner at each administration.

B. Giving Examples of Tests
Based on your experiences having taken tests over the years, try to come up with an example of each of the different types of tests listed:
1. Norm-referenced, standardized test: _____
2. Norm-referenced, non-standardized test: _____
3. Criterion-referenced, standardized test: _____
4. Criterion-referenced, non-standardized test: _____

V. Categories of Tests

Below are a number of different kinds of test categories. In small groups or as a class, write in brief definitions of each of them.

A. Ability Testing: Achievement Testing
1. Survey achievement tests:_____
2. Diagnostic tests: _____
3. Readiness tests:_____

B. Ability Testing: Aptitude Testing
1. Cognitive ability tests (mental ability tests):_____
2. Individual intelligence tests: _____
3. Neuropscyhological assessment:_____
4. Special aptitude tests: _____
5. Multiple aptitude tests: _____

C. Personality Assessment
1. Interest inventories: _____
2. Objective personality tests: _____
3. Projective tests:_____

D. Informal Assessment
1. Rating scales: _____
2. Observation:_____
3. Records and documents:_____
4. Classification methods: _____
5. Environmental assessment: _____
6. Performance-based assessment: _____

VI. Using Tests with Clients

Examine the scenarios below and discuss the kind of assessment instruments you might use in the situation. (You might want to consider the test categories from Exercise V in determining your answer.)

1. Johnny is a 12-year-old child in seventh grade. His grades have always been average, but recently his math scores have dropped considerably. In addition, he tells you that he found out not long ago that his parents are getting divorced.
2. William is 35 years old and recently separated from his wife. A few months following the separation, his wife accused him of molesting their 4-year-old child. He vehemently denies this accusation and states that she is "just saying those things in order to gain custody."
3. Judy is applying for a high-security job with the CIA. Following a background check, as a matter of course, they give her a number of assessment instruments.
4. Juanita is in lower management at a major computer firm. Her supervisor is thinking of recommending her for a promotion. Her new job would involve making quick decisions, and it requires a stable personality.
5. Twenty-four-year-old Jason is considering changing careers. He is not sure what career options are open for him and is unclear about what he likes to do. He is also unclear about what he is good at.

6. A large company is considering using tests to determine those individuals who may have severe pathology and who may be abusing drugs and alcohol. The company has a number of government contracts and is concerned about confidential material being leaked to competitors.
7. Jill's teacher has noticed that compared to all of her other abilities, Jill seems to do much worse in reading. She also noticed that her achievement test scores in reading are low compared to her other scores. She is suspecting that Jill might have a learning disability.
8. Serena was recently in a car accident and seems to be struggling with some cognitive impairment. On one hand, she seems to be able to function adequately to maintain her job, but on the other, there are clear cognitive "lapses" and some memory loss.

VII. Defining Validity
In the space provided, write a short definition of each of the types of validity listed below:
1. Face:
2. Content:
3. Criterion-related:
    a. Concurrent:
    b. Predictive:
4. Construct:
    a. Experimental:
    b. Factor analysis:
    c. Discriminant:
    d. Convergent:

VIII. Defining Reliability
In the space provided, write a short definition of each of the types of reliability listed below:
1. Test retest:

2. Parallel (equivalent or alternative forms):

3. Split-half:

4. Internal consistence (coefficient alpha, Kuder-Richardson):

IX. Evaluating a Test
A. The Passion Test
Take the "Passion Test" in Figure 12.1, and then respond to the following questions:
1. How might you show that this test is or is not valid?
2. How might you show that the test is or is not reliable?
3. What cultural assumptions are made in the test that could lead to bias? Explain.
4. What assumptions does this test make about men, women, and sexual orientation?

> **Figure 12.1: The Passion Test**
>
> **Using the following response choices, answer each item:**
> a. very true   b. somewhat true   c. a little bit true   d. not at all true
>
> 1. ___I like to have romantic dinners.
>
> 2. ___I think Jessica Alba or Matthew McConaughey is very hot.
>
> 3. ___I like to have flowers sent to me.
>
> 4. ___I prefer spicy food to bland food.
>
> 5. ___I would like to spend a week on the Riviera.
>
> 6. ___To me, romance is all in the mind.
>
> 7. ___I make love at least once a day.
>
> 8. ___I would rather have a steamy conversation than have sex.
>
> 9. ___I believe that passion is related to how much a person cares about you.
>
> 10. ___I exercise at least three times a week.

B. Examining Published Reviews about Tests

Your instructor will have students gather into groups of two or three and assign each group to one of the 10 test categories listed below. (If there are not enough students for each of the subcategories, try to have one group for each broader category.)

Tests of Educational Assessment
1. Survey battery
2. Diagnostic
3. Readiness
4. Cognitive ability tests

Cognitive Ability and Intelligence
5. Individual intelligence tests
6. Neuropsychological assessment

Career and Occupational Assessment
7. Interest inventories
8. Special aptitude and multiple aptitude tests

Clinical Assessment
9. Objective tests of personality
10. Projective personality tests

Task: In your small groups, using an online or hard copy of the *Mental Measurement Yearbook*, *Tests in Print*, or some other source that provides a thorough review of tests, obtain information about a test or tests that fit your category and respond to the following questions. Share your reviews in class:
1. Give the name of the instrument.
2. Describe the test.
3. Is the test valid? How is this shown?
4. Is the test reliable? How is this shown?
5. What evidence shows that the test is, or is not, cross-culturally fair?
6. To which population is the test geared?
7. What is the name and address of the test publisher?
8. What is the cost of the test?

X. Measures of Central Tendency and Variability

In order to make sense out of a group of scores and to understand an individual's score relative to his or her norm (peer) group, measures of central tendency and measures of variability are often used. Give a brief definition of each kind of measure of central tendency and measure of variability listed.

A. Measures of Central Tendency:
1. Mean:

2. Median:

3. Mode:

B. Measures of Variability:
1. Range:

2. Interquartile range:

3. Standard deviation:

C. Comparison of Two Normal (Bell-shaped) Curves:
Examine the differences in the bell-shaped curves depicted in Figure 12.2, and respond to the following questions:
1. Which curve has the larger standard deviation?
2. Which curve has more variability?
3. Can the means of both curves be the same?
4. If the means of both curves are the same, which curve has the largest mode?
5. If the means of both curves are the same, how can you describe the median?
6. If these tests represent scores on a test of depression, and lower scores are reflective of less depression, which group has fewer depressed individuals?
7. If these tests represent scores of aptitude as a researcher, and higher scores means more aptitude, which group has a greater number of individuals with aptitude in research?
8. If these tests represent scores on a group achievement test, is it possible to determine which group has done better?
9. What kind of general statements can you make in comparing the two curves?

Figure 12.2: Comparison of the Variability of Two Different Normal Curve Distributions

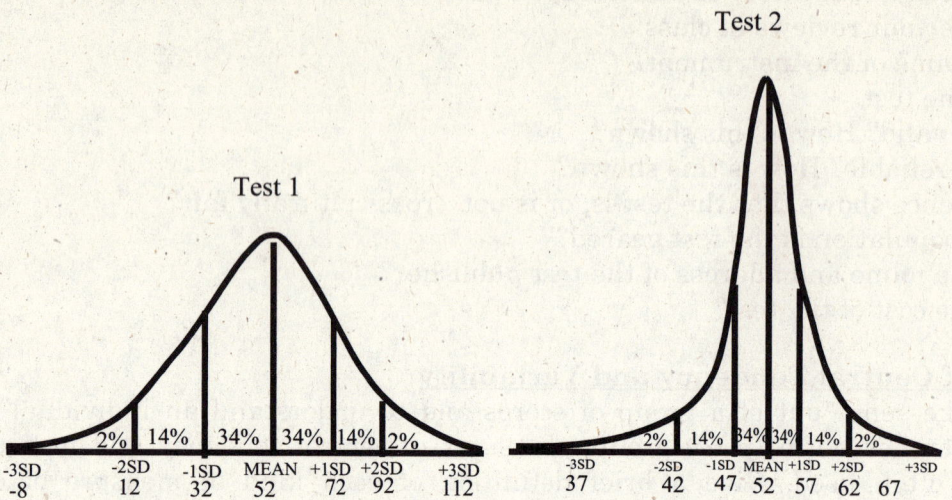

XI. Derived Scores
A number of different types of scores are used in describing an individual's test scores. Such scores are often called derived scores, some of which are listed below. Either in small groups in class, or as a homework assignment, give a brief definition of each type of derived score listed. When appropriate, list the mean and standard deviation of each derived score.
1. Percentiles
2. Stanines
3. Grade equivalents
4. Deviation IQs
5. T-scores
6. Normal curve equivalents
7. Sten scores
8. SAT/GRE-type scores
9. ACT-type scores
10. Publisher's standard scores
11. Age norms

XII. Identifying Placement on the Normal Curve of Derived Scores
Using the derived scores given below, estimate the approximate percentage of individuals who would score above and below the derived score given. If you need assistance doing this exercise, use the chart in Appendix H.
1. A percentile of 32 and a percentile of 64
2. z-scores of $-.5, -.2, +1.5, +3.2$
3. T-scores of 22, 45, 60, 68
4. DIQ scores of 48, 72, 102, 135
5. Stanines of 2, 4, 7, 9
6. Sten scores of 2, 4, 7, 9

7. SAT/GRE scores of 250, 550, 625, 780
8. ACT scores of 11, 14, 19, 24
9. NCE scores of 21, 48, 67, 89

XIII. Informal Assessment Procedures
Come up with examples of each of assessment procedure listed below. One example for each category is given:
1. Rating scales (example: student evaluation of teaching)
   Other:
2. Observation (example: observation of an acting out child in a classroom)
   Other:
3. Records and documents (example: past grades on an achievement tests)
   Other:
4. Classification methods (example: feeling word checklist)
   Environmental assessment (example: visiting client's home to assess environment)
   Other:
5. Performance-based assessment (example: graduate student portfolio)
   Other:

XIV. Familiarizing Yourself with Some Common Tests
There are literally hundreds, perhaps thousands, of tests and assessment procedures that one can consider using. However, only a few dozen tests are commonly used. For each of the commonly used tests listed in the left column, fill in the test category with which it corresponds. The possible test categories are given below. For instance, the Tennessee Self-Concept Scale is a type of objective personality test; therefore, "objective personality test" is filled in directly across from it.

Test Categories
- *Achievement tests:* survey, diagnostic, readiness
- *Aptitude tests:* individual intelligence tests, neuropsychological assessment, cognitive ability, special aptitude, multiple aptitude
- *Personality tests:* objective, projective, interest inventories
- *Informal tests:* rating scales, observation, classification system, records and personal documents, environmental assessment

1. Tennessee Self-Concept Scale   *Objective personality test*
2. The Strong   _____
3. Iowa Test of Basic Skills   _____
4. Behavior Checklist   _____
5. S.A.T./G.R.E.   _____
6. Event sampling   _____
7. Numerical scale   _____
8. Stanford-Binet   _____
9. Home visit   _____
10. Seashore Musical   _____
11. Time sampling   _____
12. General Aptitude Test Battery   _____

13. Thematic Apperception Test _____
14. Bender Gestalt II _____
15. Myers-Briggs _____
16. Gesell _____
17. California Achievement Test _____
18. Semantic Differential _____
19. Cumulative folders _____
20. Structured interview _____
21. Rorschach _____
22. WISC-IV _____
23. ASVAB _____
24. Otis-Lennon _____
25. M.M.PI.-2 _____
26. WRAT _____
27. Self-Directed Search _____
28. Kinetic Family Drawing _____
29. Situational _____
30. Genogram _____
31. Draw-a-Person _____
32. Differential Aptitude Test _____
33. California Personality Test _____
34. Key-Math _____
35. Kuder _____
36. Peabody Individual Achievement Test _____
37. Boston Process Appraoch _____
38. Coopersmith _____
39. State-Trait _____
40. Meier _____
41. Piers-Harris _____
42. Vineland Social Maturity Scale _____
43. Beck Depression Inventory _____
44. Rotter Sentence Completion _____
45. 16PF _____
46. Millon _____
47. Halstead-Reitan _____
48. Feeling Word Checklist _____

XV. Assessment of the Individual: More than Just Testing

The purpose of a client assessment is to distinguish patterns of ability or personality in order to determine an individual's general way of being in the world. The use of tests is one method of assisting an individual in understanding his or her abilities and personality. However, other methods, including the clinical interview, can add to this understanding.

A. Understanding the Clinical Interview
The clinical interview is probably the most important assessment procedure. The interview, in conjunction with tests, can tell us much about a person. Below are some broad categories of information you would want assess when conducting a clinical interview. For each of the categories, write in specific information that you might want to ask about in a clinical interview.

1. Demographic information:

2. Reason for assessment:

3. Family background:

4. Significant medical/counseling history:

5. Substance use and abuse:

6. Educational and vocational history:

7. Other pertinent information:

8. Mental status report (appearance, cognitive functioning, affect, mood):

9. DSM-IV-TR diagnosis using all five axes (note: if DSM 5 is published, use it instead):

B. Conducting a Clinical Interview
With a fellow student or another person of your choice, conduct a clinical interview. Make sure that you cover the categories listed above. Are there other categories you would also like to include? In small groups, discuss what you obtained through your interview.

C. Integrating the Clinical Interview with Other Assessment Instruments
After you have finished your clinical interview in Exercise B, consider how such an interview could be combined with tests and other assessment procedures to offer a broad picture of the individual. If your instructor wants, develop a test report that is no longer than four pages (single-spaced) based on the categories above.

XVI. Ethical, Legal, and Professional Vignettes
(The ACA's code is at www.counseling.org under "Resources"). In responding to the following, consider referring to the ACA's code.

1. During the taking of some routine tests for promotion, it is discovered that based on the results of the tests, there is a high probability that one of the employees is abusing drugs and is a pathological liar. The firm decides not to promote him and instead fires him. Is this ethical? Professional? Legal?

2. While administering a survey achievement test in the schools, a test administrator notices that a fourth grader who has been diagnosed as having attention deficit disorder with hypertension (ADHD) is "bouncing off the walls" and not able to concentrate. The test administrator asks the counselor, who is the test coordinator for the school, what she should do. The counselor says, "Just make sure he finishes the test." Is this ethical? Professional? Legal?

3. An African-American mother is concerned that her child may have an attention problem. She goes to the teacher, who supports her concerns, and they go to the assistant principal requesting testing for a possible learning problem. The mother asks if the child could be given an individual intelligence test that can screen for such problems, and the assistant principal states, "Those tests have been banned for minority students, because of concerns about cross-cultural bias." The mother says that she will give her permission for such testing, but the assistant principal says, "I'm sorry, we'll have to make do with some other tests and observation." Is this ethical? Professional? Legal?

4. A test in which there is no research to show whether it is predictive for perspective graduate students in counseling from nondominant groups is used as part of the counseling program's admission process. When challenged on this, the head of the program states that, "The test has not been proven to be biased, and we do have other criteria that we also use for admission." Is this ethical? Professional? Legal?

5. A social worker with no training in career development is giving interest inventories as she counsels individuals for career issues. Can she do this? Is this ethical? Professional? Legal?

6. A father learns that his son has obtained a low score on a self-concept inventory indicating he may have low self-esteem. The father believes that the test is bogus, walks into the school counselor's office, and demands to see the test, as well as any other records the counselor has on his son. Does the father have a right to these records?

7. A counselor routinely gives a battery of tests when beginning individual counseling with a client. After having seen a client for a few months, the counselor receives a subpoena from the court for all test records. The court wants to review the records to help decide custody of the client's children, as the client is going through a divorce. Under what circumstances, if any, can the court subpoena such records?

8. A counselor who works in the personnel office of a big company has been asked to give a series of psychological tests to help determine if any potential new employees are seriously disturbed or using drugs. The counselor tells all potential new employees that the tests are being used to "get a sense of your personality style." In light of informed consent issues, can the counselor ethically do this? Is this legal?

9. An individual who was denied employment with the FBI decides five years later to try to figure out why she was not employed. She walks into the FBI office and says, "Based on the Freedom of Information Act, I have a right to all my records, including the results of those damn personality tests you had me take." Does she have a point?

10. A counselor who has received no training in the administration and interpretation of intelligence tests decides to give the tests under supervision of a licensed school psychologist. The school psychologist helps to train the counselor and tries to ensure that the counselor is accurately administrating and interpreting the tests. They split the fee the counselor receives for the testing. Is this ethical? Professional? Legal?

11. A counselor begins to offer workshops to aid in the taking of the SATs and GREs. After researching how his participants do, he boasts in an ad that "Ninety percent of those who take my course increase their scores by 100 points." Is this ethical? Professional? Legal?

12. A court orders a suspected child abuser to go through a series of psychological tests. The suspected abuser says, "I know my rights. I can't be ordered to take any tests. There is this thing called informed consent." Is he right?

13. An individual who recently had a stroke is given a series of neuropsychological assessment procedures to assess his cognitive functioning. After completing the assessment, his employer asks him if he can have a copy because he is concerned about his job performance since the stroke. The client gives permission, in writing, to the employer to get a copy of the assessment from the examiner. Should the examiner give the assessment results to the employer? Does the employer have a right to ask about the results from the employee? What implications might the results have on the employee?
14. Your school counseling director asks all counselors to start giving self-esteem inventories to all of the students. You realize that the instrument is old and may have not shown cross-cultural fairness. You tell this to your counseling director, but she responds by saying, "We've been using it for years, and we've never had any problems—just use it." What should you do? What is your professional and ethical obligation at this point?

CHAPTER 13

MULTICULTURAL COUNSELING

I. Diversity in the World

A. Population of the World by Countries and Regions
Identify the 10 most populated countries in the world and then place them in circle on the left based on the percentage of the world they represent (42% of the world represents "all other countries"). The whole pie should equal 100%. Then, in the circle on the right, place the percentage of people in the world by the following continents: North America, South America, Europe, Africa, Asia, and Oceania. See Appendix I for the answers.

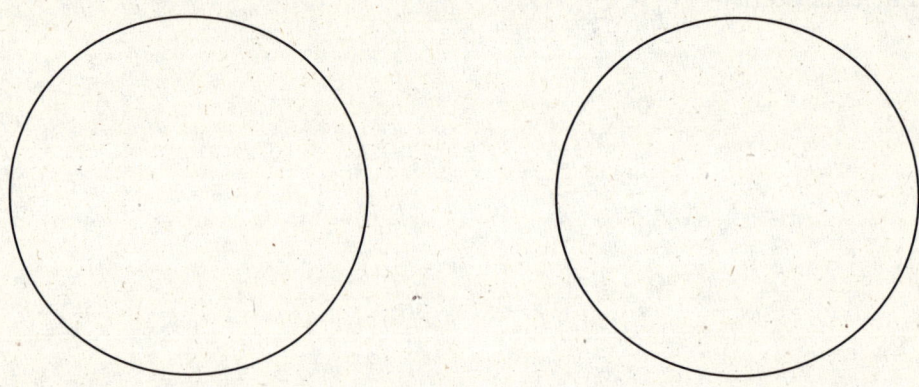

B. Select Religions of the World
Fill in the pieces of the pie on the left to represent all Christians, Buddhists, Muslims, Hindus, and Jews in the world. In addition, include a piece of the pie called "other" to represent the percentage of individuals who are agnostic, atheists, or follow other religions. When you finish with the pie on the left, represent the number of Christians as represented by Catholics, Orthodox, and Protestants in the world by filling in the pie on the right. When you are finished, turn to Appendix I to see the actual distribution.

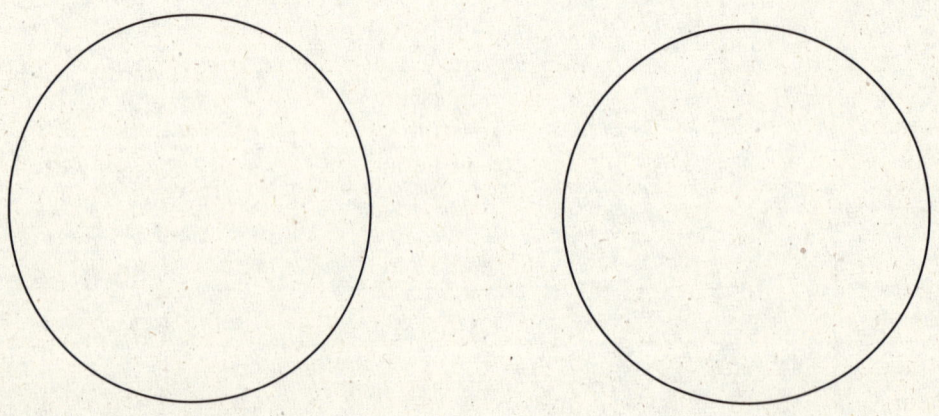

C. Diversity in the United States

Table 13.1 lists some of the ethnic, cultural, and religious groups to which Americans might belong. In the space provided, place the percentage and/or number of Americans you believe occupy each of the represented groups. Check the completed chart in Appendix I and compare your results with it.

Table 13.1 Number and Percentage of Individuals from Select Racial, Ethnic, Cultural, Religious, and Sexual Identity Backgrounds in the U.S.

Ethnicity/Race	Number (millions)	Percentage	*Religion*	Number (millions)	Percentage
White	____	____	Christian		
Black or African American	____	____	Non-Catholic	____	____
Hispanic	____	____	Catholic	____	____
Asian	____	____	Select Religious/Nonreligious Groups		
American Indian and Alaska Native	____	____	Baptist	____	____
Native Hawaiian and other Pacific Islander	____	____	Christian Generic	____	____
			Mainline Christians		
Two or More Races	____	____	(Methodist/Lutheran Episcopalian/United Church of Christ)	____	____
			Pentecostal	____	____
Sexual Orientation			Mormon	____	____
Gay		____	Jewish	____	____
Lesbian		____	Eastern Religions (e.g., Buddhist)	____	____
Gay, Lesbian, or Bisexual		____	Atheist/Agnostic		
			None	____	____

II. The Alligator River: Understanding Our Values*

First, read the alligator river story in Box 13.1. Then do Exercise A or B.

Box 13.1: Alligator River

Lovey is in a committed relationship with Fine who lives on the other side of Alligator River. Lovey wants to see Fine, but the bridge is out due to a recent flood. Lovey could try to swim across the river, but would likely be eaten by alligators. Therefore, Lovey goes to Popeye, who is the only person with a boat on the river, and asks Popeye for a ride to the other side of the river.

Popeye has always been infatuated with Lovey from a distance. Popeye has a severe speech impediment, low self-esteem, and has rarely dated. Popeye earns a meager living taking people across the river. When Lovey asks Popeye for a ride across the river Popeye states, "Lovey, I've always been infatuated with you, and I'll take you across the river if you'll make love with me." Lovey is initially disgusted and goes to a close confidant named Friend for advice. Friend states, "This is your problem, and you're going to need to work it out on your own." Lovey ponders the situation and thinks, "What the hell, I've slept with lots of people, one more won't make a difference." After they have sex, Popeye, as promised, takes Lovey across the river.

When Lovey gets to the other side of the river, out of a sense of honesty, Lovey tells Fine the whole story. Becoming enraged, Fine states, "Get out of my life, I never want to see you again." Lovey becomes distraught and seeks advice from a friend named Slug. Slug becomes infuriated and punches out Fine.

A. Examining Values as a Function of Gender and Ethnicity
Scoring Your Results: Using the grid at the end of this exercise, rate each of the five characters in the story. Place an X under number 1 and across from the name of the person you like most; then place an X under number 2 and across from the name you like second most; and so forth. Your instructor will then count up all the 1s, 2s, 3s, 4s, and 5s in the class and place them on a master grid on the board. Then, as a class, respond to the following questions:
1. What does the distribution tell you about how students in your class view individuals with differing values?
2. Based on the characters' roles, did you assume that certain characters in the story were male and others were female?
3. Consider how you might rate the characters if you changed their gender.
4. If the characters in the story were of differing ethnic, cultural, or religious backgrounds, would you have responded differently to them?
5. If you were in a helping relationship with any of the characters in the story, how would your positive and negative stereotypes affect your work with them?

B. Alternative to the above Exercise
Instead of having the class complete Exercise A, the instructor will break the class down into six groups and have each group make assumptions about the characters as noted below. Then, using the scoring instructions in Exercise A, collect the aggregate data for each of the six groups and compare the responses. (Feel free to create other groups of different gender and ethnic mixes.)
1. Group 1 (all characters are White): Lovey is female, Fine is male, Popeye is male, Friend is female, Slug is male.
2. Group 2 (all characters are a people of color; the instructor chooses the cultural group(s)): Lovey is female, Fine is male, Popeye is male, Friend is female, Slug is male.
3. Group 3 (Female characters are White, male characters are a nondominant group chosen by your instructor): Lovey is female, Fine is male, Popeye is male, Friend is female, Slug is male.
4. Group 4 (Male characters are white, Female characters are a cultural group chosen by your instructor): Lovey is female, Fine is male, Popeye is male, Friend is female, Slug is male.
5. Group 5 (all characters are female).
6. Group 6 (all characters are male).

*This exercise is adapted from the book by Simon, Howe, and Kirschenbaum (2006), *Values clarification: A handbook of practical strategies for teachers and students*. Ellington, CT: Values Realization.

	1	2	3	4	5
Lovey					
Fine					
Popeye					
Friend					
Slug					

III. Counseling Myths Questionnaire

Using the scale below, write the number to the left of each statement that best represents your view (Box 13.2). When finished, the class can discuss their varying responses. Allow different points of view to be expressed and heard. Your instructor might wish to obtain a mean and standard deviation for the class.

```
1_____2_____3_____4_____5
strongly agree    agree        no opinion       disagree      strongly disagree
```

Box 13.2:   Counseling Myths Questionnaire

1. __ Certain clients should be avoided because of their past experiences.
2. __ Cultural myths and stereotypes cannot be avoided when working with culturally different clients.
3. __ Cultural myths and stereotypes are often a reality.
4. __ Large behavioral differences exist between clients as a function of their culture.
5. __ Counselors have fewer problems when they understand their clients' backgrounds.
6. __ Counselors work best within their own cultural group.
7. __ Clients from the same ethnic background, religion, or culture have similar issues to work on.
8. __ Culturally different clients should usually be referred to counselors from the same cultural group.
9. __ Cultural differentness of client and counselor is a significant factor in the helping relationship.
10. __ Cultural variations exist regarding verbal and nonverbal communication.
11. __ Everyone is culturally different; therefore, counselors need a model that will serve all clients.
12. __ All types of social services are available for all people who desire them.
13. __ All cultures receive fair treatment in the helping relationship.
14. __ Clients from nondominant groups use profanity more often than White clients.
15. __ White clients are more likely to respond to helping interventions than non-White clients.
16. __ Generally, clients from low-income backgrounds are very difficult to help.
17. __ Many culturally different people have shown they do not trust counselors.
18. __ Family ties are extremely weak for many culturally different clients.
19. __ Value systems for many culturally different clients are inferior.
20. __ Clients from a low socioeconomic status do not trust middle-class counselors.
21. __ Sociocultural history represents the most important ingredient in the helping relationship.
22. __ Culturally different clients do not possess qualities such as boldness, initiative, and assertiveness.
23. __ Clients from nondominant groups tend not to be logical thinkers, problem solvers, or good decision makers.

> 24. ___ All helping relationships have a cross-cultural component.
> 25. ___ Religious differences are not as important as cultural differences in the helping relationship.
> 26. ___ Age differences are not as important as cultural differences in the helping relationship.
> 27. ___ Gender differences are not as important as cultural differences in the helping relationship.
> 28. ___ Sexual-orientation differences are not as important as cultural differences in the helping relationship.
>
> *Adapted with permission from Dr. Richmond Calvin, Indiana University—South Bend.

IV. Being "Other"

Your instructor will ask you to find a safe and quite space in the classroom and have you close your eyes and relax as he or she reads the following. Afterward, you will have an opportunity to discuss your experience.

1. Close your eyes, relax, and think about a time when you felt different or outside of the group or norm.

2. Slowly, begin to see, hear, feel, and smell the area around you in that memory—the people, places, time of day or night. Stay in that moment. (Pause)

3. Now move deeper into that memory. Remember, see, hear, feel, and smell what you were doing during that time. (Pause)

4. Reflect on how intensely you felt, and now feel, during that moment in your memory.

5. Now just sit in that feeling for a moment. (Pause)

6. Now please open your eyes.

7. THAT is the feeling that many people of color, gays, lesbians, transsexuals, bisexuals, and other individuals from nondominant groups experience almost every day of their lives.

*This exercise was adapted from material by Dr. Adrian S. Warren, LPC Supervisor. Her contribution is greatly appreciated.

V. Examining Our Heritage

In class, your instructor will have you form small groups of four or five. In your group, state your full name (if you're married and use your spouse's last name, include your birth name). Then discuss what you know about your name. Note such things as the origins of your last name, why you were given your first name, and any other information about your family history that is portrayed in your name. If you are not familiar with the history of your family name, you may want to ask a parent or relative and see what they know. You may want to share some of the more interesting facts you learn about one another with the whole class.

VI. Acknowledging Our Cultural/ Ethnic/Religious Affiliation
A. Who Am I?
Using Table 13.2, in the space provided, write your age, race/cultural, religious affiliation, gender, relationship status, sexual orientation, and spiritual orientation (you can leave some blank if you don't know). Then, check how often you are conscious of each characteristic. Reflect on the meaningfulness of each characteristic and how it consciously or unconsciously affects your life. Then go on to Exercise B.

	How Often Do You Think of this Group?			
Group	Every Day	Often	Sometimes	Never
Age:				
Race/Cultural Identity:				
Religion:				
Gender:				
Relationship status:				
Sexual Orientation:				
Spiritual Orientation:				

*This exercise was adapted from material by Stephanie Dailey, doctoral student at Argosy University. Her contribution is greatly appreciated.

B. Diversity in Our Midst
Using the responses to the categories (e.g., age, race, etc.) you identified in Exercise A, write them down anonymously on an index card. Then, the instructor should gather all index cards, mix them up thoroughly, and going through them one by one, write each response on the board (to maintain anonymity, the instructor should go through one characteristics at a time, and reshuffle the cards every time he or she begins a new characteristic). After all of the responses have been written on the board, examine the great diversity that exists in your classroom. Then, if you so desire, go on to Exercise C.

C. Finding out about Other Cultural Groups
After completing Exercise B, each student can anonymously write any question he or she would like answered by the diverse groups listed on the board. Your instructor will anonymously collect the questions, and, as a class, you can all help answer the questions as best you can. It is important to allow any individual to respond to the question and *not* to pressure any other individual who may have an affiliation to a specific group to become the spokesperson for that group.

VII. Interviewing a Person from another Cultural Group
Using the following questions, interview a person from a different ethnic, cultural, and/or religious/spiritual group than yours. In class, share what you learned about that person:
1. What benefits does he or she attribute to being a member of that group?
2. What drawbacks does he or she attribute to being a member of that group?
3. What history does he or she know about his or her group?
4. What are the individual's feelings concerning stereotypes of the group?
5. What prejudice has he or she experienced?
6. How would he or she feel about seeing a counselor of a differing ethnic, cultural, or religious background? Of the same background?

VIII. Experiencing Prejudice

Your instructor will have the class divide up based on some physical attribute (for example, hair color, eye color, height). In addition, your instructor will randomly pick some of these groups to be below-average, average, and above-average intelligence. Within your group, come up with stereotypes of the other groups. During class, respond to one another based on your stereotypes and on the chosen intelligence level. At the end of class, process how the experience felt.

IX. Examining the Main Values of Counseling

Column two of Table 13.2 lists the inherent values usually found in counseling relationships in the United States. Standard English is generally spoken, counselors usually believe that clients should take responsibility for themselves, and so forth. Take the cultural groups listed across the first row, or any other groups of your choice (simply place the name of the group in the top row of column six), and compare the values usually found in the counseling relationship to values you believe these cultural groups generally embrace. What differences do you notice? What can the counselor do to make the counseling relationship more amenable to the clients that you identified?

X. The Culturally Competent Counselor

First, review the Multicultural Counselor Competencies in Appendix B. Then, your instructor will break you into small groups where you will be asked to discuss your view of the effective cross-cultural counselor. What is different about this counselor as compared to a counselor who cannot work effectively with culturally different clients? Share your answers with the class, and have your instructor make a list, on the board, of the qualities of the culturally competent counselor. If you have not done Exercise XI in Chapter 3, you may want to do it now to heighten your awareness of what areas you need to work on.

Table 13.2: Focus of Counseling Relationship and Focus of Specific Cultural Groups on Select Attributes

	Usual Focus of Counseling in U.S.	Latinos/ Latinas	Muslims	Gay Men	Other?
Primary Language	Standard English				
Locus of Control/ Responsibility	High locus of control and responsibility				
Major Values	Openness, intimacy; cause and effect; analytical self-disclosure				
Mental and Physical Processes	Dichotomous; mind/body separation				
Gender Focus	Nonsexist ideals stressed				
Focus on Family	Nuclear family				
Religion	Generally neutral				

XI. Racist, Sexist, and Culturally Offensive Terms and Jokes
A. Offensive Words
Your instructor will ask all students to list every racist, sexist, or culturally offensive word or term they can think of. Write them on the board. Then, discuss the following:
1. Why do people use these terms?
2. How does each of us respond when we hear these terms?
3. What responsibility does the counseling profession have to combat the use of these terms?
4. What responsibility does each of us have toward combating the use of these terms?

B. Offensive Jokes
Your instructor will ask all students to anonymously write down racist, sexist, or culturally offensive jokes. Your instructor will then gather these and then discuss each of them with the class. Use the following questions as a guideline.
1. Why do people say these jokes?
2. What may be the origins of the jokes?
3. How does each of us respond when we hear others say such jokes?
4. What responsibility, if any, do we have to confronting people who tell such jokes?

C. Garbage In, Garbage Out
After you have finished Exercises A and B, take a piece of paper that has all of the terms and jokes on it and throw it out, symbolically getting rid of these offensive items. While throwing the items out, the class should make a commitment to combat the use of such terms and jokes by confronting those who use them.

XII. Cross-Cultural Counselor Development
A. Counselor Development of Students from Minority Groups
If you are from a nondominant group, examine Table 13.3 and try to identify the stage in which you see yourself. Reflect on what you might do to make changes in your development. When you are finished, go on to Exercise C. If you are White, go on to Exercise B.

Table 13:3: Racial/Cultural Identity Development Model

Stages Of Minority Identity Development Model (Mid)	Attitude Toward Self	Attitude Toward Others of the Same Minority	Attitude Toward Others of Different Minority	Attitude Toward Dominant Group
Stage 1— *Conformity*	Self-depreciating	Group-depreciating	Discriminatory	Group-appreciating
Stage 2— *Dissonance*	Conflict between self-depreciating and appreciating	Conflict between group-depreciating and group-appreciating	Conflict between dominant-held views of minority hierarchy and feelings of shared experience	Conflict between group-appreciating and group-depreciating
Stage 3— *Resistance and Immersion*	Self-appreciating	Group-appreciating	Conflict between feelings of empathy for other minority experiences and feelings of culturocentrism	Group-depreciating
Stage 4— *Introspection*	Concern with basis of self-appreciating	Concern with nature of unequivocal appreciating	Concern with ethnocentric basis for judging others	Concern with the basis of group-depreciation
Stage 5— *Synergetic Articulation and Awareness*	Self-appreciating	Group-appreciating	Group-appreciating	Selective appreciation

Source: *Counseling American Minorities* (6th ed.), by D. R. Atkinson (Ed.), p. 41. Copyright © 2004. The McGraw-Hill Companies. Reprinted by permission of The McGraw-Hill Companies.

B. White Counselor Development
If you are White, examine the stages of White development listed in Box 13.3. Reflect on what you can do to make changes in your development. When finished, go on to Exercise C.

C. Identity Development Discussion
Your instructor will break the class into small groups. Discuss the identity models you have reviewed, and, if you so choose, reveal your stage of identity development to others in your group. What makes you believe you are in this stage? What can increase your stage level?

> **Box 13.3: Stages of White Development**
>
> *Stage 1, Pre-exposure.* In this stage, most white graduate students show naiveté and ignorance about multicultural issues. Sometimes they believe that racism does not exist or, if it does, only to a limited degree. Racism is generally thought of as over, and students in this stage do not understand more subtle, embedded racism.
>
> *Stage 2, Exposure.* Students enter this stage when first confronted with multicultural issues. Often, this occurs when students take a course in multicultural counseling or encounter multicultural issues as a component of a class. Increasing awareness concerning how racism is embedded in society leads students in this stage to have feelings of guilt, depression with this newfound awareness, and/or anger over the current state of affairs. This stage is often highlighted by a sense of conflict between wanting to maintain majority views and the desire to uphold more humanistically oriented non-racist and non-prejudicial views.
>
> *Stage 3, Prominority/antiracism.* With movement into this stage, students often take a strong pro-minority stance, are likely to reject racist and prejudicial beliefs, and sometimes will reject their own "whiteness" in an effort to assuage the guilt felt in stage 2. Students in this stage tend to have an intense interest in diverse cultural groups and are likely to have an increasing amount of contact with individuals from different cultures.
>
> *Stage 4, Retreat to white culture.* In this stage, some white students tend to retreat into their own culture as they experience rejection from some minority individuals as they, of course, are dealing with their own identity issues. As students enter this stage, intercultural contact is ended because they feel hostile and fearful of minorities. The cozy home of the student's culture of origin is feeling quite safe at this point in time.
>
> *Stage 5, Redefinition and integration.* Students who enter this stage are developing a world view of multiculturalism and are integrating this into their identity. Such students are able to feel good about their own identity and their roots, and simultaneously have a deep appreciation of the culture of others. Students in this stage are able to expend energy toward deeply rooted structural changes in society.
>
> From Sabnani, Ponterotto, and Borodovsky (1991).

XIII. Multicultural Competence, Advocacy, and Social Justice
A. Evaluating if Your Program Attends to Multicultural Competence
After reviewing the Multicultural Counseling Competencies in Appendix B, in small groups, evaluate your counselor education program and discuss how your program does or does not foster these competencies.

B. Evaluating if Your Program Attends to Advocacy Competence
A. After reviewing the Advocacy Competencies in Appendix C, in small groups, evaluate your counselor education program and discuss how your program does or does not foster these competencies.

C. Advocacy and Social Justice vs. Traditional Counseling

Some people believe that there is little place for advocacy within the counseling relationship. For each of the situations below, consider whether you would be likely to advocate for the client in the method noted. What might be the negative and positive impact of such advocacy on the client?

1. Your client wants to obtain his GED diploma but felt demeaned when he went to his local high school to ask about the process of obtaining a GED. You decide to go with him to help empower him obtain the information.
2. You have a client with a panic disorder, and as a result, she is fearful of looking for a job. You have decided to help her identify potential jobs and go to possible job interviews with her and wait outside of the office as she interviews.
3. A female client of yours has been sexually harassed by her superior. She is fearful of reporting him. You encourage her to report him and tell her that if she allows him to continue with this behavior, he will likely harass others.
4. Using the same scenario as the one in vignette 3, this time you decide, after talking with your client, to report the client's superior yourself.
5. An African-American client tells you that the realtor he has been working with has refused to show him certain properties in mostly White neighborhoods. Your client says, "That's the way it is, and that's the way it always will be." You encourage your client to report the realtor, but he refuses. You therefore report the realtor anonymously.
6. A gay high school student you have been working with is bullied by others in his school because of his sexual orientation. Without asking for permission from your client, you decide to contact the school counselor and ask her to provide a series of workshops on understanding gay and lesbian youths and on bullying.

XIV. Identifying Counseling Needs of Clients from Nondominant Groups

Below is a list of select cultural groups. Some individuals from such groups have unique needs in the counseling relationship that are related to their culture/ethnic background. Identify one or more of the groups listed, and discuss how you think the counseling relationship might best work with individuals from that group. Feel free to add other groups to this list.

African Americans	Latinos/Latinas	Asians
Native Americans	Fundamentalist	Men
Women	Gay men	Lesbians
Bisexuals	Older people	The mentally ill
Disabled individuals	Homeless individuals	The poor
HIV-positive individuals	Transgendered people	Atheists

XV. Counseling Gays and Lesbians

Review the movie *Brokeback Mountain* or a similar movie that addresses issues of repression of homosexuality and identity development of gays and lesbians. After reviewing the video, have the class respond to the following questions:

1. What gay and lesbian stereotypes were obvious?
2. Is the "coming out" process developmental?
3. How do your beliefs about gay and lesbian marriage affect your ability to work with gay and lesbian clients?
4. What are your thoughts about gay and lesbian parenting? (Note: Some states have made it illegal for gays and lesbians to be adoptive parents.)

5. How proactive should a professional association, like the ACA or the Association of Multicultural Counseling and Development (AMCD), be in addressing issues related to gays and lesbians?
6. How proactive should you be in addressing gay and lesbian issues?
7. What counseling interventions may be unique to gays, lesbians, and bisexuals?
8. What are your thoughts about "reparative" or "conversion" therapy?
9. Discuss ACA's stance against the use of reparative therapy. Do you think a client should ever be referred for reparative therapy?
10. Other?

XVI. Gaining Knowledge about Select Groups

Interview an individual in one or more of the populations listed below, and ask the accompanying questions (and any other questions you think would be appropriate):

A. A Person from a Nondominant Group
1. When did you first realize that you were a person from a nondominant group?
2. How did you feel you "fit in" to society when you realized you were not like the majority of people?
3. Explain negative and positive experiences that you might attribute to being from a nondominant group?
4. What prejudices have you experienced?
5. What services have you been able to use due to your status as a "minority"?
6. What are your thoughts about being given services that Whites cannot obtain?
7. Overall, how do you think your ethnic/cultural group views counseling?
8. Would you, personally, see a counselor? Why or why not?

B. An Individual Who Has a Disability
1. How did you become disabled?
2. What unique experiences have you had related to your disability?
3. What prejudices have you experienced?
4. What social services have you used?
5. What social services would you like to have available?
6. Is there anything you would like to have changed about your life related to your current status?

C. A Poor Person and/or Homeless Person
1. How did you become homeless or poor?
2. What unique experiences have you had related to your current life situation?
3. What prejudices have you experienced?
4. What social services have you used?
5. What social services would you like to have available?
6. How do you make it financially day-to-day?
7. What financial resources are available to you?

D. An Individual Who Is (or Was) Chemically Dependent
1. What led you to become chemically dependent?
2. What drugs and/or alcohol do (have) you use(d)?
3. What unique experiences have you had related to your substance abuse?
4. What prejudices have you experienced?
5. What social services have you used?
6. What social services would you like to have available?
7. How do you currently expect to handle your addiction to drugs and/or alcohol?

E. An Individual Who Is HIV Positive
1. How did you become HIV positive?
2. What unique experiences have you had related to being HIV positive?
3. What prejudices have you experienced?
4. What social services have you used?
5. What social services would you like to have available?
6. What societal changes would you like to see take place relative to your HIV-positive status?

F. An Older Person
1. How do you feel about being an older person?
2. What unique experiences have you had related to your age?
3. What prejudices have you experienced?
4. What social services have you used?
5. What social services would you like to have available?
6. What attitudes related to aging would you like to see changed in society?

G. An Individual Who Struggles with Mental Illness
1. When do you first remember having to deal with your mental health problems?
2. What unique experiences have you had related to your mental illness?
3. What prejudices have you experienced?
4. What social services have you used?
5. What social services would you like to have available?
6. Has medication assisted you with your mental health problems?
7. What changes in the mental healthcare delivery system would you like to see?

XVII. Ethical, Legal, and Professional Vignettes
(The ACA's code is at www.counseling.org under "Resources"). In responding to the following, consider referring to the ACA's code.
1. Because of cross-cultural differences, you believe that your work with an Asian client has not been successful. Rather than referring the client to another counselor, you decide to read more about your client's culture in order to gain a better understanding of him. Is this ethical? Is this professional?
2. You discover some fellow students making sexist jokes. What should you do? Have you encountered such behavior? Have you acted?
3. You find some family members making ethnic/cultural slurs. What should you do? Have you encountered such behavior? Have you acted?
4. A colleague of yours identifies herself as a feminist counselor. You know that when she works with some women, she actively encourages them to leave their husbands when she discovers the husband is verbally or physically abusive. Is she acting ethically? Should you do anything?

5. You discover that a colleague of yours is telling a gay client that he is acting immorally. What should you do? Is this ethical? Professional? Legal?
6. A friend of yours advertises that she is a Christian counselor. You discover that when clients come to see her, she encourages reading parts of the Bible during sessions and tells clients they need to ask repentance for their sins. Is this ethical? Is this professional? Is this legal?
7. An African-American counselor in private practice who has expertise in a specific mental health problem decides he should only work with African-American clients. A White client who has this problem and has heard that this counselor is quite effective calls him for an appointment. The counselor refers him to someone else and tells the client he works only with African Americans. Does the African-American counselor have a responsibility to see this client? Is he acting ethically? Professionally? Legally?
8. When working with an Asian client who is not expressive of her feelings, a counselor you know pressures the client to express feelings. The counselor tells the client, "You can only get better if you express yourself." Is this counselor acting ethically? Professionally? Do you have any responsibility in this case?
9. When offering a parenting workshop to individuals who are poor, you are challenged when you tell them that "hitting a child is never okay." They tell you that you are crazy, and that sometimes a good spanking is the only thing that will get the child's attention. Do they have a point? What should you do?
10. A counselor who is seeing a client who is HIV positive discovers that his client is having sex with others without revealing his HIV status. You tell him that you have a responsibility to report him to the police. Would this be ethical? Professional? Legal?
11. A colleague of yours is working with a Latina client who states there is little hope for happiness in her marriage. The client states that her husband's attitude toward her is constantly demeaning, but that there is little she can do. After all, she tells you, it is "out of her control" and in God's hands. Your colleague tells you that she is helping the client gain autonomy and to give up the notion of "fatilismo" or that fate controls one's life—a common value held by many Latinos/Latinas. Is your colleague acting appropriately? Is there a better way for her to respond?
12. A professor of yours is a transsexual, and students in your class make jokes about him. What is your professional responsibility in this case? What thoughts do you have regarding your fellow students?
13. A colleague of yours regularly refers gay men to reparative therapy, even when they are content with their sexuality? What is your ethical and professional responsibility?
14. Based on a colleague's understanding of the research, he is against referring gay men for reparative therapy. One day, a gay man who is very depressed and upset about his sexuality asks the counselor for a referral to a reparative therapist. The colleague explains the lack of research and discusses with the client the positive and affirming aspects of being gay. The client begs for a referral, and the counselor finally gives him one. Has the counselor acted professionally? Ethically? Legally?

CHAPTER 14

SPECIALTY AREAS IN COUNSELING

I. Roles and Functions of Counselors

Below is a list of the many different settings in which you find counselors. In class or at home, pick one or more of these settings and write brief descriptions of what you think the counselor does at the setting. You may want to follow this up by accessing roles and functions from http://online.onetcenter.org/ and comparing the roles and functions listed there to the ones that you wrote. Roles and functions will also be addressed in Exercise II.

A. School Counseling
1. Elementary schools:

2. Middle schools:

3. High schools:

B. Agency and Clinical Mental Health Counseling
1. Career and employment agencies:

2. Crisis centers:

3. Community mental health centers:

4. Correctional facilities:

5. Department of social services:

6. Family service agencies:

7. Gerontological settings:

8. Group homes:

9. HMOs, PPOs, and EAPS:

10. Hospices:

11. The military and government:

12. Pastoral, religious, and spiritual counseling agencies:

13. Private practice settings:

14. Psychiatric hospitals:

15. Rehabilitation agencies:

16. Residential treatment centers:

17. Shelters for battered women:

18. Substance abuse settings:

19. Youth services programs::

C. **College Counseling**
1. Academic support services:

2. Admissions:

3. Assessment and evaluation office:

4. Career development services:

5. Commuter services:

6. Counseling centers:

7. Disability services:

8. Distance learning site directors:

9. Financial aid offices:

10. Health services:

11. Human resources:

12. Multicultural student services:

13. Office of the registrar:

14. Residence life and housing services:

15. Student activities services:

16. Women's/men's centers

II. Implementation of Roles and Functions
Your instructor will break the class into small groups representing school counselors, agency and clinical mental health counselors, and counselors who work in higher education settings. In your group, give examples of how each of the roles and functions listed below are implemented (the first item of each of the roles and functions for school counselors,

agency/mental health counselors, and counselors in higher education settings have been completed as an example). Feel free to add other descriptors as a result of your responses to Exercise I.

A. School Counselors

Today, the roles and functions of the school counselor are undergoing a paradigm shift as they begin to address various components of the American School Counseling Association (ASCA) National Model (ASCA, 2005). The model identifies four systems critical to the development of a counseling program, including the foundation, delivery, management, and accountability. In addition, four overarching themes that drive the implementation of the four systems are also highlighted by the model, including being an effective leader, advocate, collaborator, and systems change agent. Part I that follows asks you to define the four systems and their components. Part II asks you define the four themes.

Part 1. Four Systems of the ASCA National Model

In small groups, research the focus of each of these four systems and their components, and write a short definition of each of them in the space provided (1.a. is completed for you as an example).

1. *Foundation*
    a. *Beliefs and philosophy*: Describes the underlying principles that drive the program.

    b. *Mission statement*:

    c. *Standards and competencies*:

2. *Delivery*
    a. *Guidance curriculum*:

    b. *Individual student planning*:

    c. *Responsive services*:

    d. *System support*:

3. *Management*
    a. *Management agreements*:

    b. *Advisory council*:

    c. *Use of data*:

    d. *Action plans*:

    e. *Use of time*:

    f. *Calendars*:

4. _Accountability_
   a. *Results reports*:

   b. *Performance standards*:

   c. *Program audit*:

Part 2: Four Themes of the ASCA National Model

Having the knowledge and skills to be an effective leader, advocate, collaborator, and systems change agent is critical to being an effective school counselor, and have been identified in the National Model as overarching themes that affect the successful implementation of the four systems just discussed. Within your small groups, define each of these important roles:

1. _Leader:_

2. _Advocacy:_

3. _Collaboration and teaming:_

4. _Systems change:_

B. Agency and Clinical Mental Health Counselors
Part 1. Common Roles

Agency and mental health counselors find themselves in a number of roles. Some of the more common ones are listed below. In your small group, write down some of the tasks such a counselor might do in these roles (item 1 is completed for you as an example):

1. _Case manager:_ understanding client needs, creating treatment plans, and follow through on treatment goals, paperwork, evaluation, follow-up, billing, time management, and so forth

2. _Appraiser of client needs:_

3. _Counselor:_

4. _Consultant:_

5. _Crisis responder:_

6. _Supervisor:_

7. _Supervisee:_

Part 2. Other Roles
Agency and mental health counselors often find themselves in a vast array of other roles. In your small group, write down some of the tasks such a counselor might do in the following roles (Southern Regional Education Board, 1969):
1. *Outreach worker:*

2. *Broker:*

3. *Advocate:*

4. *Evaluator:*

5. *Teacher/educator:*

6. *Behavior changer:*

7. *Mobilizer:*

8. *Community planner:*

9. *Caregiver:*

10. *Data manager:*

11. *Administrator:*

12. *Clinical assistant:*

C. Counselors in Higher Education Setting
Delworth and Hanson (1991; Komives & Woodward, 2003) have identified four roles that counselors in higher education often take on, including counselor, educator, campus ecology manager, and administrator. These roles have a number of functions. In your small group, define each of the roles and then note how they address the many items related to these roles as listed below:
1. *Counselor*
   a. *Role model to students*: The counselor is a powerful person in a student's life, and behaviors are consciously and unconsciously taken on by students who work with the counselor.

   b. *Direct support to students:*

   c. *Providing preventive psychological programs:*

   d. *Making referrals to mental health experts:*

   e. *Requesting psychological expertise from clinicians:*

   f. *Advocating for change in the system to foster student growth:*

2. *Educator*
   a. *Advisor*:

   b. *Mentor*:

   c. *Curriculum builder/instructor*:

   d. *Evaluator-assessor*:

   e. *Scholar-researcher*:

3. *The campus ecology manager*
   a. *Physical setting*:

   b. *Human aggregates*:

   c. *Organizational structure and dynamics*:

   d. *Perceptual or constructed environments*:

4. *The administrator*
   a. *Students*:

   b. *Services and programs*:

   c. *Structure*:

   d. *Staff*:

   e. *Funding sources and other resources*:

III. Implementing Roles and Functions Using a Developmental Perspective

Counselors have always prided themselves on using developmental models when addressing client concerns (e.g., Erikson, 1963, 1980, 1982; Chickering, 1969, Chickering & Reisser, 1993; see Table 14.1 and Box 14.1). Your instructor will divide the class into small groups based on students' proposed specialty area of concentration. After you are in your small group, use one of the developmental models given, or a developmental model of your choice, and address the tasks in Exercise A, B, or C.

A. Developmental School Counseling

In your group, use Erikson's model (Table 14.1) or another model of your choosing to show how you would use the ASCA National Model when addressing student concerns. Address each of the four systems and four themes when implementing your developmental guidance and counseling program (see Exercise 2.A). Be specific.

Table 14.1: Erickson's Psychosocial Stages of Development

Stage	Name of Stage with Ages	Virtue of Stage	Description of Stage
1	Trust vs. Mistrust (Birth-1)	Hope	In this stage, the infant is building a sense of trust or mistrust, which can be facilitated by significant others' ability to provide a sense of psychological safety to the infant.
2	Autonomy vs. Shame and Doubt (1-2)	Will	Here, the toddler explores the environment and is beginning to gain control over his or her body. Significant others can either promote or inhibit the child's newfound abilities and facilitate the development of autonomy or shame and doubt.
3	Initiative vs. Guilt (3-5)	Purpose	As physical and intellectual growth continues and exploration of the environment increases, a sense of initiative or guilt can be developed by significant others who are either encouraging or discouraging of the child's physical and intellectual curiosity.
4	Industry vs. Inferiority (6-11)	Competence	An increased sense of what the child is good at, especially relative to his or her peers, can either be reinforced or negated by significant others (e.g., parents, teachers, peers), leading to feeling worthwhile feelings, or being discouraged by others, which leads to feeling inferior.
5	Identity vs. Role Confusion (Adolescence)	Fidelity	Positive role models and experiences can lead to increased understanding of the temperament, values, interests, and abilities that define one's sense of self. Negative role models and limited experiences will lead to role confusion.
6	Intimacy vs. Isolation (Early Adulthood)	Love	A good sense of self and self-understanding leads to the ability to form intimate relationships that are highlighted by mutually supporting relationships that encourage individuality with interdependency. Otherwise, the young adult feels isolated.
7	Generativity vs. Stagnation (Middle Adulthood)	Caring	Healthy development in this stage is highlighted by concern for others and for future generations. This individual is able to maintain a productive and responsible lifestyle and can find meaning through work, volunteerism, parenting, and/or community activities. Otherwise, the adult feels stagnant.
8	Ego Integrity vs. Despair (Later Life)	Wisdom	The older adult who examines his or her life either feels a sense of fulfillment or despair. Successfully mastering the developmental tasks from the preceding stages will lead to a sense of integrity for the individual.

B. Developmental Agency/Mental Health Counseling

In your group, use Erikson's model (Table 14.1) or another model of your choosing to show how you would use the roles and functions of community agency/mental health counselors noted earlier when addressing client concerns. Address each of the common roles as well as most or all of the additional roles listed (see Exercise 2.B). Be specific.

C. Developmental Student Affairs Counseling

In your group, use Chickering's model (Box 14.1) or another model of your choosing to show how you would address student concerns. In your response, address each of the four roles identified earlier for student affairs practitioners (see Exercise 2.C). Be specific.

Box 14.1: Chickering's Seven Vectors

Chickering believed that students struggle with seven vectors when attending college and graduate school (Chickering, 1969; Chickering & Reisser, 1993). They included each of the following:

1. *Achieving competence.* Chickering believed that each student's ability to successfully develop his or her intellectual, physical, and interpersonal competence is crucial during the college years and that such growth ultimately leads one to a sense of self-worth.
2. *Managing emotions.* As students develop into adulthood, they increasingly struggle with finding ways of managing emotions, especially anger and emotions related to their sexuality, both of which become ever more salient in the college years. The task for students is to establish new, more mature ways of managing all of their emotions.
3. *Developing autonomy.* The developing college student is increasingly faced with issues of autonomy as he or she disengages from his or her family of origin and develops a separate sense of self.
4. *Establishing identity.* As students become autonomous, self-sufficient adults, they are better able to understand their intellectual, physical, and interpersonal competence and strive to more effectively manage their emotions. In this process, students begin to examine who they are within these domains and establish a sense of identity.
5. *Freeing interpersonal relationships.* As individuals increasingly become more aware of their own identity, they are better able to form relationships with others and ultimately become more tolerant of differences.
6. *Developing purpose.* Perhaps one of the most important vectors, developing purpose relates to how individuals make meaning out of their lives. Deciding what is worth striving for can only be accomplished if an individual has a clear sense of who he or she is—in other words, if he or she has established an identity.
7. *Developing integrity.* This last vector has to do with one's ability to develop a value system governed by a well-thought-out belief system. Such a value system is the basis for moral action in the developing adult.

IV. Contrasting the Focus of Counselors in Different Specialty Areas

Using Figure 14.1, contrast the different foci of the counseling relationships of school counselors, agency/clinical mental health counselors, and counselors in higher education settings. Do this by placing an S to represent school counselors, an A to represent agency/mental health counselors, and an H to represent counselors in higher education settings directly on each of the attributes listed in Figure 14.1. In some cases, you might wish to place more than one letter, if you believe that the attribute may be expressed differently in various settings within a specialty area. For instance, for the attribute "Short-term/Long-term," you might believe that in some higher education settings, one might be more likely to use short-term counseling approaches, while in other higher education settings, long-term approaches are more the norm. After you are finished, see if there are major differences among the three specialty areas and if the specialty area is more likely to be practicing guidance, counseling, or psychotherapy.

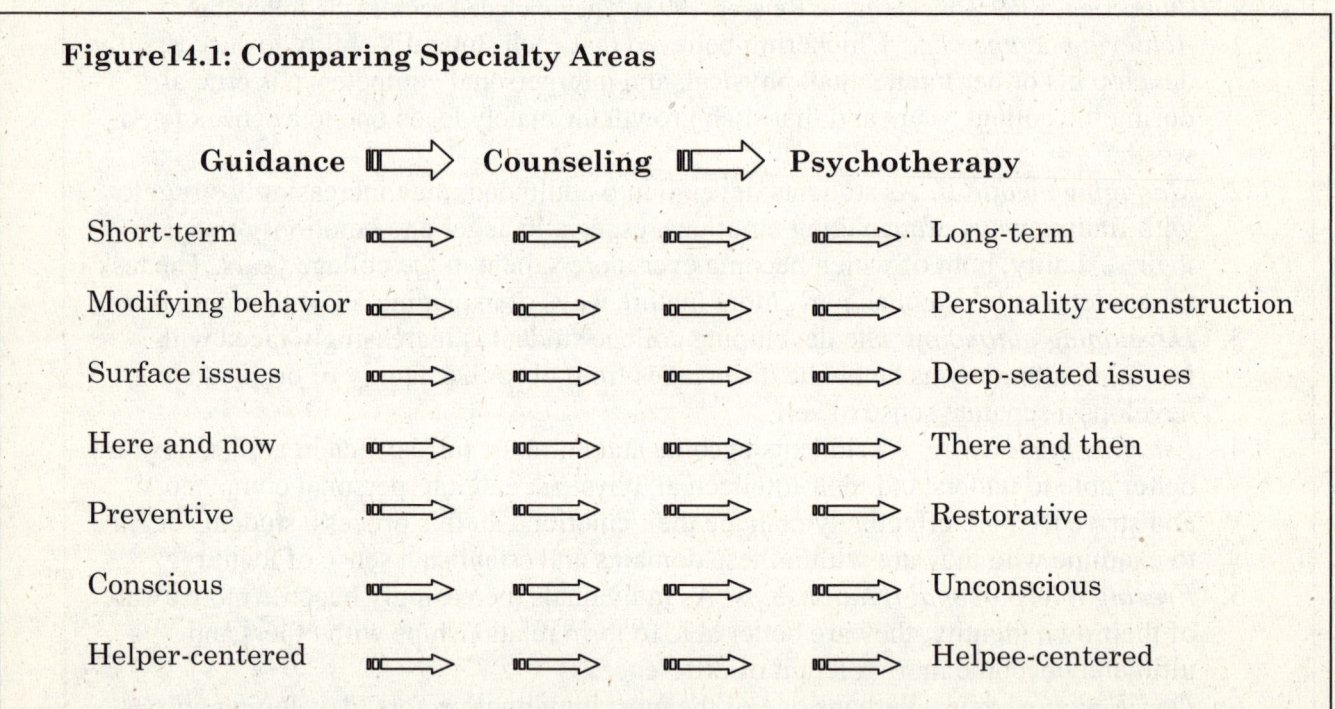

V. The Use of Counseling Theories in Different Settings

After completing Exercise IV, consider the kinds of counseling theories that would be most amenable to the settings we have examined. For instance, if you have found that a setting mostly focuses on "guidance," you might be more likely to use a theoretical approach that is developmental in nature and/or short term. Make a list of the theory and the setting and the justification why you would use the theory you chose (You may want to examine Appendix D to review descriptions of the different theories). Share in small groups or in class.

VI. Ethical, Legal, and Professional Vignettes.

In responding to the following, consider referring to the ACA's code at www.counseling.org (under "Resources").

A. School Counseling

1. A student with whom you are working reveals to you that she has been seriously beaten by her mother. You immediately go to your principal, who tells you not to report this to Child Protective Services because there are no visible bruises. What should you do? Do you have an ethical and/or legal obligation to report the situation to Child Protective Services?
2. You are working with a child who has very low self-esteem. The parent of the child comes to see you and asks to know specifics about what the child is revealing in counseling. You tell the parent that what is talked about in counseling is confidential. Have you responded in an ethical and professional manner? Is this legal?
3. A teenager with whom you are working reveals to you that she is sexually active and not using contraception. You encourage her to use contraception and tell her how and where she can obtain various forms of birth control. Is this ethical? Professional? Legal?
4. You discover that one of the students you are counseling is pregnant. You counsel her on the various options, including abortion. Is this ethical? Professional? Legal?
5. You have been asked to sit on a Child Study Team (Special Education Team) for a student. You discover that the student is the son of one of your neighbors. Should you continue to be a member of this team? Would this be ethical? Professional? Legal?
6. You are working with a student whose grades have dropped precipitously. You discover that the student's parents have separated, and the student is depressed. The student's teacher comes up to you and wants to know why the student is suddenly doing so poorly in her classes. What should you say?
7. You're doing group counseling with fifth-grade female students. The students tell you about some friends of theirs, who are in the same school, who were engaged in same-sex sexual activity the week before at a sleepover. What should you do?

B. Agency/Mental Health Counseling

8. A neighbor of yours comes to the local community mental health center where you are working, seeking counseling. He has been referred to you by another counselor. You tell your supervisor that this person is your neighbor. After you reveal to your supervisor that you rarely, if ever, have contact with him and know nothing about his life, the supervisor tells you to go ahead and be his counselor. Is this ethical? Professional?
9. After having worked as a school counselor for a number of years, you apply for a job as an outpatient therapist at a mental health center. Is this ethical? Professional? Are there any requirements that you need to have met to make the shift from one setting to another?
10. Because you don't believe in the use of diagnosis, when asked to make a diagnosis at your agency, you tend to minimize clients' problems and give the least stigmatizing diagnosis. Is this ethical? Professional? Legal?
11. Despite research indicating that medication in conjunction with therapy is more effective than either medication or therapy alone for depressed clients, a colleague of yours refuses to refer clients for medication. Is this ethical? Professional? Legal? Should you say anything to your colleague?

12. A fellow student of yours tells you that she wants to become credentialed as a school counselor, but really hopes to get a job in agency counseling. She figures that if she doesn't find a job in an agency, she can fall back on her credential in school counseling. She therefore finished the school counseling track in the counseling program. Is this ethical? Professional? Should you do anything?

C. Counseling in Higher Education Settings

13. You are counseling a college student for depression. One day, you receive a call from the student's parents, wanting to know why their daughter is in counseling. What should you say? Are you obligated to keep the information gained during counseling confidential? Are you obligated to reveal any information to the parents?
14. While working in residence life, a counselor discovers, through an informal counseling session with a student, the names of other students who are using drugs in the residence hall. The counselor has those students suspended. Has the counselor acted ethically? Professionally? Legally?
15. While working at a college counseling center, you are informed by the supervisor of the center to stop seeing a client because the client has used up the maximum number of sessions available to students. You believe the client is suicidal. You also know that the client has no insurance coverage for mental health services, so it would be difficult for him to find a referral. You tell this to your supervisor, but he says, "I told you to stop seeing him. Find a referral!" You decide to secretly see the client. Have you acted ethically? Professionally? Do you have any other options?
16. You are asked to run a series of training sessions for faculty on multicultural sensitivity. You discover during your training that one faculty member is overtly racist and is likely to treat minorities differentially in class. You decide to tell the administration about what you have discovered. Have you acted ethically? Professionally?
17. You believe that the administration of the college where you work is not attending to issues of hazing and the use of alcohol. You are concerned that a student could be seriously harmed or even die. You say something to the administration, but they ignore your complaints. You decide to go to the local newspaper with your concerns. Have you acted ethically? Professionally? Were there any other alternatives?

CHAPTER 15

GOING TO GRADUATE SCHOOL, GETTING A JOB

I. How Did You Get Here?
If you have been accepted into a graduate school, or have made a decision about which school you would like to go to, make a list of why you decided to choose that school. Also, make a second list of the factors you think should be considered in choosing a graduate school. Share your list in small groups or with the whole class.

II. Choosing a Graduate School
If you have not yet chosen a graduate school to attend, or if you are considering going on for advanced training, you might want to examine the items below when deciding which school to attend. Compare the lists made by students in Exercise I with the list below. Are there additional items you think should be included to the list below? The Graduate Degree Exploration Worksheet in Appendix J (McCurdy, 1998) covers the material on this list and more, to assist you in making this challenging decision. It will also help you to identify the best programs for you to consider applying.

1. Program accreditation [e.g., CACREP, APA, NASW]
2. Client emphasis
3. Philosophical orientation
4. Counseling specialties offered
5. Degree requirements
6. Correlation of degree requirements with certification requirements
7. Degree granted
8. Entry requirements
9. Location
10. Size
11. Faculty-student ratio
12. Location of field experience
13. Placement of recent graduates
14. Cost
15. Availability of scholarships, fellowships, and loans
16. Diversity of faculty and of students

III. Applying to Graduate School
A. Items to Consider When Applying
After completing the Graduate Degree Exploration Worksheet in Appendix J, review your results in small groups. Discuss the importance of your responses to each of the items on the worksheet. Pay close attention to the following when applying to graduate school:

1. Meeting deadlines
2. Completing forms
3. Taking a cognitive ability test (e.g., GREs)
4. Writing an essay
5. Interviewing
6. Interviewing
7. Submitting a résumé
8. Preparing a portfolio
9. Reapplying if denied

B. Comparing Résumés and Portfolios
Bring to class your résumé and/or portfolio, and compare its strengths and weaknesses with other students. See Exercise VII for items you might consider including in your résumé.

C. Writing an Essay
In class, your instructor will disseminate one or more essay questions and have you write practice essays for graduate school. This can be completed either at home or in class. Compare your essays in class. Check for content, grammar, and spelling. If completed at home, check for appearance and neatness.

IV. Finding a Graduate School
Either on your own or in small groups, obtain one or more of the books or visit one or more of the websites listed below. Then compare and contrast the various types of graduate programs that interest you. These resources will assist you in completing the Graduate Degree Exploration Worksheet (see Appendix J).

- *Master's and doctoral programs in counseling*:
  Council for Accreditation of Counseling and Related Educational Programs
  1001 North Fairfax Street, Suite 510
  Alexandria, VA 22314
  Phone: (703) 535-5990
  Website: www.cacrep.org
  Related association: American Counseling Association

  Counselor Preparation: Programs, Faculty, Trends (12th ed.) (2008).
  Authors: Schweiger, W., Henderson, D., Clawson, T., Collins, D., & Nuckolls, M.
  Routledge, c/o Taylor & Francis, Inc.
  7625 Empire Drive
  Florence, Kentucky 41042-2919
  Phone: (800) 634-7064
  Website: www.routledge.com/
  Email: orders@taylorandfrancis.com

- *Doctoral programs in counseling and clinical psychology:*
  American Psychological Association (APA)
  750 First Street NE
  Washington, DC 20002
  Graduate and Postdoctoral Education
  Phone: (202) 336-5979
  Website: www.apa.org/education/grad/index.aspx
  Related association: American Psychological Association (www.apa.org)

- *Master's programs in rehabilitation counseling:*
  Council on Rehabilitation Education
  1699 Woodfield Rd., Suite 300
  Schauburg, IL 60173
  Phone: (847) 944-1345
  Website site: www.core-rehab.org

Email: sdenys@cpcredentialing.com
Related association: Am. Rehabilitation Counseling Association (www.arcaweb.org)
National Rehabilitation Counseling Association (http://nrca-net.org)

- ***Master's programs in marriage and family therapy***:
  <u>Commission on Accreditation for Marriage and Family Therapy Education</u>
  112 South Alfred Street
  Alexandria, VA 22314-3061
  Phone: (703) 838-9808
  Website: www.aamfte.org (then click "education and training" and then "accreditation")
  Related association: Am. Association for Marriage and Family Therapy (www.aamft.org)

- ***Clinical pastoral programs:***
  <u>Association for Clinical Pastoral Education, Inc.</u>
  1549 Clairmont Road, Suite 103
  Decatur, GA 30033
  Phone: (404) 320-1472
  Website: www.acpe.edu

- ***Master's programs in social work:***
  <u>Council on Social Work Education</u>
  1725 Duke St., Suite 500
  Alexandria, VA 22314
  Phone: (703) 683-8080
  Website: www.cswe.org/Accreditation.aspx
  Related associations: Council on Social Work Education (www.cswe.org)
  National Association of Social Workers (www.naswdc.org)

- ***Master's programs in art therapy:***
  <u>American Art Therapy Association</u>
  225 North Fairfax Street
  Alexandria, VA 22314
  Phone: (888) 290-0878
  Website: www.americanarttherapyassociation.org/aata-educational-programs.html
  Related association: American Art Therapy Association (www.arttherapy.org)

V. Finding a Job

In small groups, discuss the importance of each of the following when applying to graduate school:
1. Networking
2. Going on informational interviews
3. Responding to ads in professional publications
4. Interviewing at national conferences
5. Using college and job placement services
6. Looking in the newspaper
7. Being on counseling "listservs" and related social-networking forums

VI. Role-play Interviewing

In small groups, your instructor will have you practice role-play interviews for graduate school or for a job. One student will play an employer or faculty member while a second student will play an interviewee. In addition, two students can be observers and offer feedback. The observers should pay particular attention to the following:
1. The nonverbals of the interviewee
2. The ability of the interviewee to respond fully to questions
3. The ability to demonstrate knowledge in response to questions asked
4. The enthusiasm of the interviewee
5. Knowledge of basic counseling skills and values of the counselor
6. Knowledge of professional counseling organizations
7. Desire to pursue knowledge and scholarly activities
8. Knowledge of the setting to which the interviewee is applying
9. The tendency of the interviewee to be positive
10. The attire of the interviewee

VII. Creating a Résumé

Below are some do's and don'ts of résumé writing. Please note there are a number of good books on résumés such as *Amazing Résumés* (Bright & Earl, 2009) or *Best Résumés for College Students and New Grads* (Kursmark, 2006). In addition, today, there are some great websites to help you build a terrific résumé.

A. Some Do's and Don'ts of Résumés

1. Incorporate all significant jobs into your résumé, including those that may not be counseling related (any job shows your depth of experience)

2. Include as many of the following sections that may be relevant:
    a. Education
    b. Work experience
    c. Professional memberships
    d. Conference attendance
    e. Research interest
    f. Publications
    g. Honors and awards
    h. Service to the profession
    i. Service to the community
    j. Names of references
    k. Other?

3. Consider the following:
    a. Do brag about yourself.
    b. Do check your spelling and use good grammar.
    c. Do make sure your résumé looks good, is readable, and is correct.
    d. Do tailor your résumé to the requirements of the program or job being pursued.
    e. Don't sell yourself short.
    f. Don't lie or bend the truth.
    g. Don't use gender-bias words or phrases.
    h. Don't be overly concerned about length. Whatever you decide the length your résumé needs to be, make sure it is not hard on the eyes of the reader.

    i. Don't include an objective if it might say something that could eliminate you from the pool of candidates (e.g., saying you're interested in working with children might exclude you from a job that includes working with adults).
    j. Don't make the résumé too wordy or too chaotic.
    k. Don't add detail that could have you eliminated from the selection process (e.g., your age).
    l. Don't feel like you have to follow any of the advice given to you about how to develop your résumé, including this list of do's and don'ts. Most of all, do feel comfortable with your résumé.

B. Assessing Your Résumé

Bring in a copy of your résumé, and after reviewing the do's and don'ts listed above, divide into small groups to give each other some feedback.

VIII. Creating a Portfolio

Portfolios are paper or electronic folders that contain a wide range of information that a person can use when applying for a job or graduate school (Cobia, 2005; Barnes, Clark, & Thull, 2003). Some examples of items that might be included:

    a. A résumé

    b. Transcripts or videos of the student's work with clients (clients' identities are hidden)

    c. Supervisor's assessment of the student's work

    d. A paper that highlights the student's view of human nature

    e. Examples of how to build a multicultural environment at a setting

    f. Ways that the student shows a commitment to the counseling profession

    g. A test report written by the student

    h. A major project developed school counseling

Develop a portfolio and bring it to class. In small groups, have students review each others' portfolios and identify their strengths and weaknesses.

IX. Ethical, Legal, and Professional Vignettes

In responding to the following, consider referring to the ACA's code (located at www.counseling.org, under "Resources").

1. A fellow student shows you his résumé. On it, he has stated that he has expertise in working in addictions. You know that he has only taken one course in addictions and has no work experience in that area. Is this ethical? Professional? What obligation do you have, if any, to confront him?
2. A student you know has stated on his résumé that he has been the lead researcher on a manuscript. You know that he has been assisting a professor, and it is unlikely that his name will even appear on the article. Is this ethical? Professional? What obligation do you have, if any, to confront him?
3. In developing a portfolio, a student you know has included a paper as her own that

was written by a number of students. How should you handle this situation?

4. A student you know intends to apply to a doctoral program in counseling. You have gotten to know this student fairly well as he has attended the master's degree program with you. You believe that this student has serious emotional problems and that it would be a mistake if, at this point in time, he was admitted to graduate school. What should you do, if anything?

5. You have learned that a graduate school to which you have applied has different admission standards for candidates from nondominant groups than candidates who are White. Is this ethical? Professional? Legal? Do you have any obligation in this situation to do anything?

6. You discover that an employer who has recently hired you has, in very subtle and probably unconscious ways, consistently not hired individuals from nondominant groups over the years. Is this ethical? Professional? Legal? What obligation do you have, if any, to do something?

7. You find out that in writing an essay for graduate school, a fellow student has had an editor review the essay. Is this ethical? Professional? What obligation do you have, if any, to do something?

8. You find out that in writing an essay for graduate school, a fellow student has misrepresented her credentials. Is this ethical? Professional? What obligation do you have, if any, to do something?

9. You have just graduated from a master's program that has applied for CACREP accreditation. After graduating, the program becomes accredited, and you learn that a student who graduated with you has stated on her resume that she has graduated from a CACREP-accredited institution. Is this ethical? Professional? What obligation do you have, if any, to do something?

10. A professor of yours has encouraged you not to apply to graduate school because she states, "You won't be able to handle the research." You decide to apply anyway. After applying, you discover that this same professor had an informal conversation with a colleague she knows at the school to which you applied and encouraged this colleague to not accept you. Is this ethical? Professional? Legal? What obligation do you have, if any, to do something?

REFERENCES

American Counseling Association. (2005). *Code of ethics*. Retrieved from http://www.counseling.org/Resources/CodeOfEthics/TP/Home/CT2.aspx

American School Counseling Association. (2005). *The ASCA National Model: A framework for school counseling programs* (2nd ed.). Arlington, VA: Author

American Psychiatric Association. (2000). *Diagnostic and statistical manual of mental disorders* (4th ed., text revision). Washington, DC: Author

Atkinson, D. R. (2004). *Counseling American minorities* (6th ed.). New York: McGraw Hill

Barnes, P., Clark, P., & Thull, B. (2003, November). Web-based digital portfolios and counselor supervision. *Journal of Technology in Counseling, 3*(1). Retrieved from http://jtc.colstate.edu/vol3_1/Barnes/Barnes.htm

Bertalanffy, L. von. (1968). *General systems theory*. New York: Braziller

Best, J. W., & Kahn, J. V. (2006). *Research in education* (10th ed.). Boston: Allyn & Bacon

Black, D., Gates, G., Sanders, S., & Taylor, L. (2000). Demographics of the gay and lesbian population in the United Sates: Evidence from available systematic data sources. *Demography, 37*(2), 139-154

Borders, L. D., & Brown, L. L. (2005). *The handbook of counseling supervision*. Mahwah, NJ: Lawrence Erlbaum Associates

Bright, J., & Earl, J. (2009). *Amazing résumés: What employers want to see—and how to say it* (2nd ed.). Indianapolis, IN: JIST Works

Cameron, S., & turtle-song, i. (2002). Learning to write case notes using the SOAP format. *Journal of Counseling & Development, 80*(3), 286-92

Campbell, D. T., & Stanley, J. C. (1963). *Experimental and quasi-experimental designs for research*. Chicago: Rand McNally

Cashwell, C. S. (1994). *Interpersonal process recall*. Retrieved from ERIC database (ED 372342)

Center for Disease Control. (2002). *Key statistics from the National Survey of Family Growth*. Retrieved from www.cdc.gov/nchs/nsfg/abc_list_s.htm

Chickering, A. W. (1969). *Education and identity*. San Francisco: Jossey-Bass

Chickering, A. W., & Reisser, L. (1993). *Education and identity* (2nd ed.). San Francisco: Jossey-Bass

Christensen, T. M., & Brumfield, K. A. (2010). Phenomenological designs: The philosophy of phenomenological research. In C. J. Sheperis, J. C. Young, & M. H. Daniels (Eds.), *Counseling research: Quantitative, qualitative, and mixed methods* (pp. 135-149). Upper Saddle River, NJ: Pearson

Cobia, C. D., Carney, J. S., Buckhalt, J. A., Middleton, R. A., Shannon, D. M., Trippany, R., & Kunkel, E. (2005). The doctoral portfolio: Centerpiece of a comprehensive system of evaluation. *Counselor Education and Supervision, 44*(4), 242-254

Conyne, R. K., Crowell, J. L., & Newmeyer, M. D. (2008). *Group techniques: How to use them more purposefully*, Upper Saddle River, NJ: Pearson/Merrill Prentice Hall

Cook, T. D., & Campbell, D. T. (1979). *Quasi-experimentation: Design and analysis issues for field settings.* Chicago: Rand McNally

Cooper, S. (2003). College counseling centers as internal organizational consultants to universities. *Consulting Psychology Journal: Practice and Research, 55*(4), 230-238. doi: 10.1037/1061-4087.55.4.230

Delworth, U., & Hanson, G. (Eds.). (1991). *Student services* (2nd ed.). San Francisco: Jossey-Bass

Dougherty, A. M. (2009). *Psychological consultation and collaboration in school and community settings* (5th ed.). Belmont, CA: Brooks/Cole

Erikson, E. (1963). *Childhood and society.* New York: W. W. Norton.

Erikson, E. (1980). *Identity and the life cycle.* New York: W. W. Norton

Erikson, E. H. (1982). *The life cycle completed.* New York: W. W. Norton

Fowler, J. W. (1976). Stages in faith: The structural-developmental approach. In T. C. Hennessy (Ed.), *Values & Moral Development* (pp. 173-211). New York: Paulist Press

Fowler, J. W. (1991). The vocation of faith developmental theory. In J. W. Fowler, K. E. Nipkow, & F. Schweitzer (Eds.), *Stages of faith and religious development: Implications for church, education, and society* (pp. 19-37). New York: Crossroad Publishing

Fowler, J. W. (1995). *Stages of faith: The psychology of human development and the quest for meaning.* New York: Harper & Row

Fowler, J. W. (2000). *Becoming adult, becoming Christian: Adult development and Christian faith* (rev. ed.). San Francisco: Jossey-Bass

Gilligan, C. (1982). *In a different voice.* Cambridge, MA: Harvard University Press

Gilleard, C. & Higgs, P. (2007). The third age and the baby boomers: Two approaches to the social structuring of later life. *International Joural of Ageing & Later Life, 2*(2), 13-30

Gottfredson, G. D., Holland, J. L., & Ogawa, D. K. (1996). *Dictionary of Holland occupational codes*. Odessa, FL: Psychological Assessment Resources

Greenhaus, J. H., Callanan, G. A., & Godhsalk, V. M. (2010). *Career management* (4th ed.). Thousand Oaks, CA: Sage Publications

Gysbers, N. C., Heppner, M. J., & Johnston, J. A. (2009). *Career counseling: Contexts, processes, and techniques* (3rd ed.). Alexandria, VA: American Counseling Association

Harris-Bowlsbey, J., Spivack, J. D., & Lisansky, R. S. (1991). *Take hold of your future* (Leader's Manual) (2nd ed.). Iowa City, IA: American College Testing Program

Holland, J. L. (1973). *Making vocational choices: A theory of career*. Englewood Cliffs, NJ: Prentice Hall

Holland, J. L., & Gottfredson, G. D. (1976). Using a topology of persons and environments to explain careers: Some extensions and clarifications. *Counseling Psychologist, 6*, 20-29

Hutchison, B., & Niles, S. G. (2009). Career development theories. In I. Marini, & M. A. Stebnicki (Eds.). *The professional counselor's desk reference* (pp. 467-476). New York: Springer Publishing Company

Idol, L., Nevin, A., & Paolucci-Whitcomb, P. (2000). *Collaborative consultation* (3rd ed.). Austin, TX: Pro-Ed

Kagan, N. (1980). Influencing human interaction Eighteen years with IPR. In A. I. Hess (Ed.), *Psychotherapy supervision: Theory, research, and practice* (pp. 262-283). New York: Wiley

Kagan, N., & Kagan, N. I. (1997). Interpersonal process recall: Influencing human interaction. In C. E. Watkins, (Ed.). *Handbook of Psychotherapy Supervision* (pp. 296-309). New York: John Wiley

Kampwirth, T. J. (2006). *Collaborative consultation in the schools: Effective practices for students with learning and behavior problems* (3rd ed.). Upper Saddle River, NJ: Pearson

Kaplan, D. M., Kocet, M. M., Cottone, R., Glosoff, H.L., Miranti, J. G., Mol, E. C., Tavrydas, M. L. (2009). New mandates and imperatives in the revised "ACA Code of Ethics." *Journal of Counseling & Development, 87*(2), 241-256

Kegan, R. (1982). *The evolving self.* Cambridge, MA: Harvard University Press

Kegan, R. (1994). *In over our heads.* Cambridge, MA: Harvard University Press

Kohlberg, L. (1969). *Stages in the development of moral thought and action.* New York: Holt, Rinehart & Winston

Kohlberg, L. (1984). *The psychology of moral development: The nature and validity of moral stages.* San Francisco: Harper & Row

Komives, S. R., & Woodward, D. B. (Eds.). (2003). Part five: Essential competencies and techniques. In S. R. Komives & D. B. Woodward, *Student services: A handbook for the profession* (4th ed., pp. 421-422). San Francisco: Jossey-Bass

Kosmin, B. A., & Keysar, A. (2008). *American Religious Identification Survey.* Hartford, CO: Trinity College

Kuhn, T. S. (1962). *The structure of scientific revolutions.* Chicago: University of Chicago Press

Kursmark, L. M. (2006). *Best résumés for college students and new grads: Jump-start your career* (2nd ed.). Indianapolis, IN: JIST Works

Lent, R. W. (2005). A social cognitive view of career development and counseling. In S. D. Brown & R. W. Lent (Eds.). *Career development and counseling: Putting theory and research to work* (pp. 101-127). New York: John Wiley

McCurdy, K. G. (1998, July). Should you get your Ph.D.? *Counseling Today.* Alexandria, VA: American Counseling Association

McMillan, J. H., & Schumacher, S. (2010). *Research in education: Evidence-based inquiry* (7th ed.). Boston: Allyn & Bacon

Myers, J., & Sweeney, T. J. (2008). Wellness counseling: The evidence base and practice. *Journal of Counseling and Development, 86*, p. 482-493.

Neukrug, E., & Fawcett, R. C. (2010). *Essentials of testing and assessment: A practical guide for counselors, social workers, and psychologists* (2nd ed.). Belmont, CA: Brooks/Cole

Neukrug, E. (2011). *The world of the counselor* (4th ed.). Belmont, CA: Brooks/Cole

Neukrug, E., & Milliken, T. (2012). Counselors' perceptions of ethical behaviors. *Journal of Counseling and Development*, 89, 206-216.

Patton, W., & McIlveen, P. (2009). Practice and research in career counseling and development—2008. *The Career Development Quarterly, 58*(2), 118-161

Peterson, G. W., Sampson, J. P., & Reardon, R. C. (1991). *Career development and services: A cognitive approach*. Pacific Grove, CA: Brooks/Cole

Religious Tolerance. *Female genital mutilation (FGM) in Africa, the Middle East, and Far East*. Retrieved from http://www.religioustolerance.org/fem_cirm1.htm

Roysircar, G., Arredondo, P., Fuertes, J. N., Ponterotto, J. G., & Toporek, R. L. (Eds). (2003). *Multicultural counseling competencies 2003: Association for Multicultural Counseling and Development*. Alexandria, VA: Association for Multicultural Counseling and Development

Sabnani, H. B., Ponterotto, J. G., & Borodovsky, L. G. (1991). White racial identity development and cross-cultural counselor training: A stage model. *The Counseling Psychologist, 19*(1), 76-102

Schein, R. (1969). *Process consultation: Its role in organization development*. Reading, MA: Addison-Wesley

Schein, R. (1999). *Process consultation revisited: Building the helping relationship*. Reading, MA: Addison-Wesley

Schultheiss, D. E. P. (2007). The emergence of a relational cultural paradigm for vocational psychology. *International Journal for Educational and Vocational Guidance, 7*, 191–201. doi: 10.1007/s10775-007-9123-7

Shadish, W. R., Cook, T. D., & Campbell, D. T. (2002). *Experimental and quasi-experimental designs for generalized causal inference*. Boston: Hougton Miflin

Simon, S. B., Howe, L. W., & Kirschenbaum, H. W. (2006). *Values clarification: A handbook of practical strategies for teachers and students* (rev. ed.). Ellington, CT: Values Realization

Southern Regional Educational Board (1969). *Roles and functions for different levels of mental health workers*. Atlanta, GA: Author

Stoltenberg, C. D., & Delworth, U. (1987). *Supervising counselors and therapists*. San Francisco: Jossey-Bass

Stoltenberg, C. D., McNeil, B., & Delworth, U. (1998). *IDM supervision*. San Francisco: Jossey-Bass

Stoltenberg, C. (2005). Enhancing professional competence through developmental approaches to supervision. *American Psychologist, 60*(8), 857-864

Super, D. E., & Hall, D. T. (1978). Career development: Person, position, and process. *Counseling Psychologist, 1*, 2-9

Super, D. E., Savickas, M. L., & Super, C. M. (1996) Life-span, life-space approach to careers. In D. Brown, L. Brooks, & Associates (Eds.), *Career choice and development* (3rd ed., Chapter 5). San Francisco: Jossey-Bass

Toporek, R. L., & Lewis, J. A., & Crethar, H. C. (2009). Promoting systemic change through the ACA advocacy competencies. *Journal of Counseling and Development, 87,* 260-268

United States Census Bureau. (2009). *Annual Estimates of the Resident Population by Sex, Race, and Hispanic Origin for the United States: April 1, 2000 to July 1, 2009* (NC-EST2009-03). Retrieved from http://www.census.gov/popest/national/asrh/NC-EST2009-srh.html

Watzlawick, P., Weakland, J. H., & Fisch, R. (1974). *Change: Principles of problem formulation and problem resolution.* New York: Horton

World Health Organization. (2010). *Female genital mutilation and other harmful practices.* Retrieved from http://www.who.int/reproductivehealth/topics/fgm/overview/en/index.html

Yalom, I. D., & Leszca, M. (2005). *The theory and practice of group psychotherapy* (5th ed.). Cambridge, MA: Perseus Books

APPENDIX A

PERCEPTIONS OF ETHICAL CONDUCT

The following statements describe a variety of helper behaviors. Examining each statement from the role of a helper, in **Column I** write "**E**" if you think the behavior is **E**thical or "**U**" if you think the behavior is **U**nethical. In **Column II**, rate how strongly you feel about your response in Column I (1 = not very strongly through 10 = very strongly). The first item is an example of how to respond. This person believes the statement to be Ethical ("E") and feels quite strongly that the behavior is ethical as you can see by the score of "8."

Col. I	Col. II	ITEM
E	8	1. Hugging a client
		2. Accepting a client's decision to commit suicide
		3. Viewing your client's personal webpage (e.g., MySpace, Facebook, blog) without informing your client
		4. Not reporting when you suspect that your client is being abused by his or her spouse
		5. Pressuring a client to receive needed services
		6. Withholding information about a minor client despite a parent's request for information
		7. Based on personal preference, accepting clients who are only male or only female
		8. Breaking confidentiality if the client is threatening harm to self
		9. Not allowing clients to view their records (excluding case notes)
		10. Engaging in a professional counseling relationship with a friend
		11. Guaranteeing confidentiality for couples and families
		12. Breaking the law to protect your client's rights
		13. Keeping client records on your office computer
		14. Counseling clients from a different culture with little or no cross-cultural training
		15. Based on personal preference, accepting clients only from specific cultural groups
		16. Treating homosexuality as a pathology
		17. Sharing confidential client information with your administrative supervisor
		18. Sharing confidential client information with a colleague who is not your supervisor
		19. Referring a client due to interpersonal conflicts between you and your client
		20. Being an advocate for clients

			21. Trying to persuade your client to *not* have an abortion even though she wants to
			22. Using techniques that are not theory or research based
			23. Revealing confidential information if a client is deceased
			24. Publicly advocating for a controversial cause
			25. Accepting a gift from a client that's worth more than $25
			26. Counseling a pregnant teenager without parental consent
			27. Having clients address you by your first name
			28. Refraining from making a diagnosis to protect a client from a third party (e.g., employer who might demote a client)
			29. Revealing a client's record to the spouse of a client without the client's permission
			30. Counseling a terminally ill client about end-of-life decisions including suicide
			31. Engaging in a professional counseling relationship with a colleague who works with you
			32. Using an interpreter when a client's primary language is different from yours
			33. Referring a client, unhappy with his or her homosexuality, for "reparative therapy" (therapy focused on converting sexual identity from homosexual to heterosexual)
			34. Encouraging a client's autonomy and self-determination
			35. Reporting a colleague's unethical conduct without first consulting with the colleague
			36. Kissing a client as a friendly gesture (e.g., greeting)
			37. Telling your client you are angry at him or her
			38. Keeping client records in an unlocked file cabinet
			39. Consoling your client by touching him or her (e.g., placing your hand on his or her shoulder)
			40. Engaging in a dual relationship (e.g., your client is also your child's teacher)
			41. When counseling an elderly client, not reporting suspected abuse of that client
			42. Stating you are licensed when you are in the process of obtaining your license
			43. Becoming sexually involved with a person your client knows well
			44. Not offering a professional disclosure statement
			45. Not informing clients of their legal rights (e.g., HIPAA, FERPA, confidentiality)
			46. When counseling a child, not reporting suspected abuse of that client
			47. Seeing a minor client without parental consent
			48. Attending a client's wedding, graduation ceremony, or other formal ceremony
			49. Providing services to an undocumented worker (sometimes called illegal immigrant)

		50. Referring a client who is satisfied with his or her homosexuality for "reparative therapy"
		51. Giving a gift worth more than $25 to a client
		52. Sharing confidential client information with your spouse/significant other
		53. Telling your client you are attracted to him or her
		54. Setting your fee higher for clients with insurance than for those without
		55. Making a diagnosis based on DSM-IV-TR
		56. Guaranteeing confidentiality for group members
		57. Lending money to your client
		58. Providing counseling over the Internet
		59. Trying to change your client's values
		60. Not allowing clients to view your case notes about them
		61. Terminating the counseling relationship without warning
		62. Charging for individual counseling while seeing all members of a family
		63. Becoming sexually involved with a former client (at least 5 years after the counseling relationship ended)
		64. Engaging in a helping relationship with a client (e.g., individual counseling) while the client is in another helping relationship (e.g., family counseling) without contacting the other counselor
		65. Not participating in continuing education after obtaining your degree
		66. Bartering (accepting goods or services) for counseling services
		67. Accepting a client when you have not had training in his or her presenting problem
		68. Not being a member of a professional association in counseling
		69. Not having malpractice coverage (on your own or by your agency/setting)
		70. While completing one's dissertation, using the title "Ph.D. Candidate" in clinical practice
		71. Selling a product to your client that is related to the counseling relationship (e.g., book, audiotape, etc.)
		72. Attempting to persuade your client to adopt a religious conviction you hold
		73. Making grandiose statements about your expertise
		74. Implying that a certification is the same as a license
		75. Not revealing the limits of confidentiality to your client
		76. Not having a plan to transfer your clients should you become incapacitated
		77. Self-disclosing to a client

APPENDIX B

MULTICULTURAL COUNSELING COMPETENCIES

I. Counselor Awareness of Own Cultural Values and Biases

A. Attitudes and Beliefs

1. Culturally skilled counselors believe that cultural self-awareness and sensitivity to one's own cultural heritage is essential.

2. Culturally skilled counselors are aware of how their own cultural background and experiences have influenced attitudes, values, and biases about psychological processes.

3. Culturally skilled counselors are able to recognize the limits of their multicultural competency and expertise.

4. Culturally skilled counselors recognize their sources of discomfort with differences that exist between themselves and clients in terms of race, ethnicity and culture.

B. Knowledge

1. Culturally skilled counselors have specific knowledge about their own racial and cultural heritage and how it personally and professionally affects their definitions and biases of normality/abnormality and the process of counseling.

2. Culturally skilled counselors possess knowledge and understanding about how oppression, racism, discrimination, and stereotyping affect them personally and in their work. This allows individuals to acknowledge their own racist attitudes, beliefs, and feelings. Although this standard applies to all groups, for White counselors it may mean that they understand how they may have directly or indirectly benefited from individual, institutional, and cultural racism as outlined in White identity development models.

3. Culturally skilled counselors possess knowledge about their social impact upon others. They are knowledgeable about communication style differences, how their style may clash with or foster the counseling process with persons of color or others different from themselves based on the A, B and C, Dimensions, and how to anticipate the impact it may have on others.

C. Skills

1. Culturally skilled counselors seek out educational, consultative, and training experiences to improve their understanding and effectiveness in working with culturally different populations. Being able to recognize the limits of their competencies, they (a) seek consultation, (b) seek further training or education, (c) refer out to more qualified individuals or resources, or (d) engage in a combination of these.

2. Culturally skilled counselors are constantly seeking to understand themselves as racial and cultural beings and are actively seeking a non racist identity.

II. Counselor Awareness of Client's Worldview
A. Attitudes and Beliefs
1. Culturally skilled counselors are aware of their negative and positive emotional reactions toward other racial and ethnic groups that may prove detrimental to the counseling relationship. They are willing to contrast their own beliefs and attitudes with those of their culturally different clients in a nonjudgmental fashion.

2. Culturally skilled counselors are aware of their stereotypes and preconceived notions that they may hold toward other racial and ethnic minority groups.

B. Knowledge
1. Culturally skilled counselors possess specific knowledge and information about the particular group with which they are working. They are aware of the life experiences, cultural heritage, and historical background of their culturally different clients. This particular competency is strongly linked to the "minority identity development models" available in the literature.

2. Culturally skilled counselors understand how race, culture, ethnicity, and so forth may affect personality formation, vocational choices, manifestation of psychological disorders, help seeking behavior, and the appropriateness or inappropriateness of counseling approaches.

3. Culturally skilled counselors understand and have knowledge about sociopolitical influences that impinge upon the life of racial and ethnic minorities. Immigration issues, poverty, racism, stereotyping, and powerlessness may impact self esteem and self concept in the counseling process.

C. Skills
1. Culturally skilled counselors should familiarize themselves with relevant research and the latest findings regarding mental health and mental disorders that affect various ethnic and racial groups. They should actively seek out educational experiences that enrich their knowledge, understanding, and cross-cultural skills for more effective counseling behavior.

2. Culturally skilled counselors become actively involved with minority individuals outside the counseling setting (e.g., community events, social and political functions, celebrations, friendships, neighborhood groups, and so forth) so that their perspective of minorities is more than an academic or helping exercise.

III. Culturally Appropriate Intervention Strategies
A. Beliefs and Attitudes
1. Culturally skilled counselors respect clients' religious and/ or spiritual beliefs and values, including attributions and taboos, because they affect worldview, psychosocial functioning, and expressions of distress.

2. Culturally skilled counselors respect indigenous helping practices and respect help~iving networks among communities of color.

3. Culturally skilled counselors value bilingualism and do not view another language as an impediment to counseling (monolingualism may be the culprit).

B. Knowledge

1. Culturally skilled counselors have a clear and explicit knowledge and understanding of the generic characteristics of counseling and therapy (culture bound, class bound, and monolingual) and how they may clash with the cultural values of various cultural groups.

2. Culturally skilled counselors are aware of institutional barriers that prevent minorities from using mental health services.

3. Culturally skilled counselors have knowledge of the potential bias in assessment instruments and use procedures and interpret findings keeping in mind the cultural and linguistic characteristics of the clients.

4. Culturally skilled counselors have knowledge of family structures, hierarchies, values, and beliefs from various cultural perspectives. They are knowledgeable about the community where a particular cultural group may reside and the resources in the community.

5. Culturally skilled counselors should be aware of relevant discriminatory practices at the social and community level that may be affecting the psychological welfare of the population being served.

C. Skills

1. Culturally skilled counselors are able to engage in a variety of verbal and nonverbal helping responses. They are able to send and receive both verbal and nonverbal messages accurately and appropriately. They are not tied down to only one method or approach to helping, but recognize that helping styles and approaches may be culture bound. When they sense that their helping style is limited and potentially inappropriate, they can anticipate and modify it.

2. Culturally skilled counselors are able to exercise institutional intervention skills on behalf of their clients. They can help clients determine whether a "problem" stems from racism or bias in others (the concept of healthy paranoia) so that clients do not inappropriately personalize problems.

3. Culturally skilled counselors are not averse to seeking consultation with traditional healers or religious and spiritual leaders and practitioners in the treatment of culturally different clients when appropriate.

4. Culturally skilled counselors take responsibility for interacting in the language requested by the client and, if not feasible, make appropriate referrals. A serious problem arises when the linguistic skills of the counselor do not match the language of the client. This being the case, counselors should (a) seek a translator with cultural knowledge and appropriate professional background or (b) refer to a knowledgeable and competent bilingual counselor.

5. Culturally skilled counselors have training and expertise in the use of traditional assessment and testing instruments. They not only understand the technical aspects of the instruments but are also aware of the cultural limitations. This allows them to use test instruments for the welfare of culturally different clients.

6. Culturally skilled counselors should attend to as well as work to eliminate biases, prejudices, and discriminatory contexts in conducting evaluations and providing interventions, and should develop sensitivity to issues of oppression, sexism, heterosexism, elitism and racism.

7. Culturally skilled counselors take responsibility for educating their clients to the processes of psychological intervention, such as goals, expectations, legal rights, and the counselor's orientation.

Source: Arredondo, P., Toporek, M. S., Brown, S., Jones, J., Locke, D. C., Sanchez, J. & Stadler, H. (1996). Operationalization of the multicultural counseling competencies. Alexandria, VA: Association of Multicultural Counseling and Development. Retrieved from http://www.amcdaca.org/amcd/competencies.pdf

APPENDIX C

ADVOCACY COMPETENCIES

Client/Student Empowerment
- An advocacy orientation involves not only systems change interventions but also the implementation of empowerment strategies in direct counseling.
- Advocacy-oriented counselors recognize the impact of social, political, economic, and cultural factors on human development.
- They also help their clients and students understand their own lives in context. This lays the groundwork for self-advocacy.

Empowerment Counselor Competencies
In direct interventions, the counselor is able to:
1. Identify strengths and resources of clients and students.
2. Identify the social, political, economic, and cultural factors that affect the client/student.
3. Recognize the signs indicating that an individual's behaviors and concerns reflect responses to systemic or internalized oppression.
4. At an appropriate development level, help the individual identify the external barriers that affect his or her development.
5. Train students and clients in self-advocacy skills.
6. Help students and clients develop self-advocacy action plans.
7. Assist students and clients in carrying out action plans.

Client/Student Advocacy
- When counselors become aware of external factors that act as barriers to an individual's development, they may choose to respond through advocacy.
- The client/student advocate role is especially significant when individuals or vulnerable groups lack access to needed services.

Client/Student Advocacy Counselor Competencies
In environmental interventions on behalf of clients and students, the counselor is able to:
8. Negotiate relevant services and education systems on behalf of clients and students.
9. Help clients and students gain access to needed resources.
10. Identify barriers to the well-being of individuals and vulnerable groups.
11. Develop an initial plan of action for confronting these barriers.
12. Identify potential allies for confronting the barriers.
13. Carry out the plan of action.

Community Collaboration
- Their ongoing work with people gives counselors a unique awareness of recurring themes. Counselors are often among the first to become aware of specific difficulties in the environment.
- Advocacy-oriented counselors often choose to respond to such challenges by alerting existing organizations that are already working for change and that might have an interest in the issue at hand.

- In these situations, the counselor's primary role is as an ally. Counselors can also be helpful to organizations by making available to them our particular skills: interpersonal relations, communications, training, and research.

Community Collaboration Counselor Competencies
14. Identify environmental factors that impinge upon students' and clients' development.
15. Alert community or school groups with common concerns related to the issue.
16. Develop alliances with groups working for change.
17. Use effective listening skills to gain understanding of the group's goals.
18. Identify the strengths and resources that the group members bring to the process of systemic change.
19. Communicate recognition of and respect for these strengths and resources.
20. Identify and offer the skills that the counselor can bring to the collaboration.
21. Assess the effect of counselor's interaction with the community.

Systems Advocacy
- When counselors identify systemic factors that act as barriers to their students' or clients' development, they often wish that they could change the environment and prevent some of the problems that they see every day.
- Regardless of the specific target of change, the processes for altering the status quo have common qualities. Change is a process that requires vision, persistence, leadership, collaboration, systems analysis, and strong data. In many situations, a counselor is the right person to take leadership.

Systems Advocacy Counselor Competencies
In exerting systems-change leadership at the school or community level, the advocacy-oriented
counselor is able to:
22. Identify environmental factors impinging on students' or clients' development
23. Provide and interpret data to show the urgency for change.
24. In collaboration with other stakeholders, develop a vision to guide change.
25. Analyze the sources of political power and social influence within the system.
26. Develop a step-by-step plan for implementing the change process.
27. Develop a plan for dealing with probable responses to change.
28. Recognize and deal with resistance.
29. Assess the effect of counselor's advocacy efforts on the system and constituents.

Public Information
- Across settings, specialties, and theoretical perspectives, professional counselors share knowledge of human development and expertise in communication.
- These qualities make it possible for advocacy-oriented counselors to awaken the general public to macro-systemic issues regarding human dignity

Public Information Counselor Competencies
In informing the public about the role of environmental factors in human development, the advocacy oriented counselor is able to:
30. Recognize the impact of oppression and other barriers to healthy development.
31. Identify environmental factors that are protective of healthy development.
32. Prepare written and multi-media materials that provide clear explanations of the role of specific environmental factors in human development.
33. Communicate information in ways that are ethical and appropriate for the target population.
34. Disseminate information through a variety of media.
35. Identify and collaborate with other professionals who are involved in disseminating public information.
36. Assess the influence of public information efforts undertaken by the counselor.

Social/Political Advocacy
- Counselors regularly act as change agents in the systems that affect their own students and clients most directly. This experience often leads toward the recognition that some of the concerns they have addressed affected people in a much larger arena.
- When this happens, counselors use their skills to carry out social/political advocacy.

Social/Political Advocacy Counselor Competencies
In influencing public policy in a large, public arena, the advocacy-oriented counselor is able to:
37. Distinguish those problems that can best be resolved through social/political action.
38. Identify the appropriate mechanisms and avenues for addressing these problems.
39. Seek out and join with potential allies.
40. Support existing alliances for change.
41. With allies, prepare convincing data and rationales for change.
42. With allies, lobby legislators and other policy makers.
43. Maintain open dialogue with communities and clients to ensure that the social/political advocacy is consistent with the initial goals.

Source: American Counseling Association (n.d.). Advocacy competencies. Retrieved from http://www.counseling.org/Resources/Competencies/Advocacy_Competencies.pdf

APPENDIX D

DESCRIPTIONS OF THEORETICAL ORIENTATIONS AND CONCEPTUAL ORIENTATIONS

Theoretical Orientations

Psychoanalysis. Developed by Sigmund Freud, psychoanalysis suggests that instincts, such as hunger, thirst, survival, aggression, and sex, are very strong motivators of behavior. The satisfaction of instincts is mostly an unconscious process, and defense mechanisms are developed to help manage our instincts. Because we are in a constant and mostly unconscious struggle to satisfy our instincts, psychoanalysts believe that happiness is elusive. Early child-rearing practices are responsible for how we manage our defenses and for normal or abnormal personality development. The fact that early childhood experiences forms personality and that our behaviors are mostly dictated by the unconscious lends a sense of determinism to this approach.

Analytical Psychology. Analytical psychology was developed by Carl Jung, who believed that psychological symptoms represent a desire to regain lost parts of self, as well as parts that have never been revealed to consciousness, so that the person can become whole. Analytical therapists believe that we have primitive or primordial images that interact with repressed material to cause "complexes." We inherit these images, or archetypes, and they provide the psyche with its tendency to perceive the world in certain ways that we identify as human. In addition, we are born with the mental functions of sensation–intuition and thinking–feeling, which affect our perceptions and whose relative strengths are affected by child-rearing patterns. We are also born with a tendency to be extraverted (outgoing) or introverted (observer; inward).

Individual Psychology. Developed by Alfred Adler, individual psychology suggests that early childhood experiences and the memories of those experiences result in our character or personality. If early experiences and the memories of them enhance our innate abilities and characteristics, we will have a tendency to move toward wholeness, completion, and perfection. However, a person's response to early feelings of inferiority can result in the creation of private logic and compensatory behaviors that lead toward maladaptive or neurotic behaviors. Although early experiences influence the development of personality, education and therapy can be effective in helping a person change.

Behavior Therapy. Developed by B. F. Skinner, John Wolpe, Albert Bandura, Ivan Pavlov, and others, behavior therapy is based on classical conditioning, operant conditioning, and social learning (or modeling), which suggest that how individuals are conditioned affects their personality development. They believe that conditioning is very complex and can happen in subtle ways. By carefully analyzing how behaviors are conditioned, one can understand why an individual exhibits certain behaviors and develop goals to eliminate undesirable behaviors while reinforcing new desirable behaviors.

Rational Emotive Behavior Therapy (REBT). Developed by Albert Ellis, REBT suggests that we are born with the potential for rational or irrational thinking, and it is the belief about an event that is responsible for one's reaction to the event, not the event itself. Beliefs about an event can be rational or irrational, with irrational thinking leading to emotional distress, dysfunctional behaviors, and criticism of self and others. Although individuals have a tendency to sustain the type of thinking they previously learned, irrational thinking can be challenged and individuals can adopt rational thinking if given the opportunity through counseling.

Cognitive Therapy. Developed by Aaron "Tim" Beck, cognitive therapy suggests that we are born with a predisposition toward certain emotional disorders that reveals itself under stressful conditions. Cognitive therapists also believe that genetics, biological factors, and experiences combine to produce specific core beliefs that are responsible for automatic thoughts (fleeting thoughts about what we perceive and experience), which result in a set of behaviors, feelings, and physiological responses. By understanding one's cognitive processes (e.g., core beliefs, automatic thoughts), one can address and change automatic thoughts and core beliefs that lead to dysfunctional behaviors and distressful feelings.

Reality Therapy. Developed by William Glasser, reality therapy suggests that we are born with five needs—survival, love and belonging, power, freedom, and fun—which can only be satisfied in the present. Reality therapists believe that we have a "quality world" that contains pictures in our mind of the people, things, and beliefs most important to meeting our needs. We make choices based on these pictures, although we can only choose actions and thoughts; feelings and our physiology result from those choices. At any point in one's life, one can evaluate one's behaviors, thoughts, feelings, and physiology, and make new choices. Language we use reflects the kinds of choices we have made.

Existential Therapy. Developed by Viktor Frankl, Rollo May, and others, existential therapy states that we are born into a world that has no inherent meaning or purpose, that we all struggle with the basic questions of what it is to be human, and that we alone can create our own meaning and purpose. Existential therapists believe that we all have the ability to live authentically and experience fully, but sometimes avoid such an existence out of our fears of looking squarely at how we are making meaning in our lives. They state that meaningfulness, as well as a limited sense of freedom, comes through consciousness and the choices we make.

Person-Centered Counseling. Carl Rogers founded this approach, which states that we have an inborn actualizing tendency that lends direction to our lives as we attempt to reach our full potential. However, this tendency is sometimes thwarted as individuals act in ways in which significant others want them to act due to the individual's desire to be loved and regarded by those significant others. This results in the creation of an incongruent self. Anxiety and related symptoms are a signal that the person is acting in a nongenuine way and not living fully. Being around people who are real, empathic, and show positive regard can help individuals become real.

Gestalt Therapy. Founded by Fritz Perls, Gestalt therapy suggests that we are born with the capacity to embrace an infinite number of personality dimensions. With the mind, body, and soul operating in unison, from birth, the individual is in a constant state of need identification and need fulfillment. However, parental dictates, social mores, and peer norms can prevent a person from attaining a need and results in defenses that block the experiencing of needs. Gestalt therapy highlights the importance of accessing one's experience because the "now" of experience = awareness = reality. Experiencing allows one to break free from defenses and live a saner life.

Narrative Therapy. Narrative therapy, developed by Michael White, suggests that reality is a social construction and that each person's reality is organized and maintained through his or her narrative or language discourse. Within this context, values held by those in power are often disseminated through language and become the norms against which individuals compare themselves. Therefore, problems individuals have, including mental disorders, are a function of problem-saturated stories or narratives people have in their lives, and these are created through the individual's social discourse. However, new, preferred stories can be generated.

Solution-Focused Brief Therapy. Steve de Shazer and Insoo Kim Berg, two founders of solution-focused brief therapy, suggested that problems are the result of language passed down by families, culture, and society, and dialogues between people. Therefore, pathology, in all practical purposes, is not inherently found within the person, as is professed by many therapies that describe structures that affect functioning (e.g., id, ego, self-actualizing tendency). Believing there is no objective reality, they suggest that individuals can find exceptions to their problems and build on those exceptions to find new ways of living in the world. They suggest that change can occur in fewer than six sessions, and that extended therapy is often detrimental.

Description of Broad Conceptual Orientations

Psychodynamic Approaches. (e.g., psychoanalysis, analytical therapy, and individual psychology). Developed near the beginning of the 20th century but maintaining widespread popularity today, psychodynamic approaches vary considerably but contain some common elements. For instance, they all suggest that an unconscious and a conscious affect the functioning of the person in some deeply personal and "dynamic" ways. They all look at early child-rearing practices as being important in the development of personality. They all believe that examining the past, and the dynamic interaction of the past with conscious and unconscious factors, are important in the therapeutic process. Although these approaches have tended to be long term, in recent years, some have been adapted and used in relatively brief treatment modality formats.

Cognitive–Behavioral Approaches (e.g., behavior therapy, rational emotive behavior therapy (REBT), cognitive therapy, and reality therapy). Cognitive–behavioral approaches look at how cognitions and/or behaviors affect personality development, behaviors, and emotional states. All of these approaches believe that cognitions and/or behaviors have been learned and can be relearned. They tend to spend a limited amount of time examining the past, as they focus more on how present cognitions and behaviors affect the individual's feelings, thoughts, actions, and physiological responses. They all believe that after identifying problematic behaviors and/or cognitions, one can choose, replace, or reinforce new cognitions and behaviors that result in more effective functioning. These approaches tend to be shorter than the psychodynamic or existential–humanistic approaches.

Existential–Humanistic Approaches (e.g., existential therapy, Gestalt therapy, and person-centered counseling). Loosely based on the philosophies of existentialism and phenomenology, these approaches were particularly prevalent during the latter part of the 20th century but continue to be widely used today. Existentialism examines the kinds of choices one makes to develop meaning and purpose in life, and, from a psychotherapeutic perspective, suggests that people can choose new ways of living at any point in their lives. Phenomenology is the belief that each person's reality is unique and that to understand the person, you must hear how that person has come to make sense of his or her world. These approaches tend to focus on the "here and now" and gently challenge clients to make new choices in their lives. Although generally shorter term than the psychodynamic approaches, these therapies tend to be longer term than the cognitive–behavioral approaches.

Post-Modern Approaches (e.g., narrative therapy and solution-focused brief therapy). Narrative therapy and solution-focused brief therapy are recent additions to the therapeutic milieu and are based on the philosophies of social constructivism and post-modernism. Social constructivism suggests that individuals construct meaning in their lives from the discourses they have with others and the language that is used in their culture and in society. Post-modernism suggests that all reality should be questioned. Those with this philosophy even doubt many of the basic assumptions of past popular therapies, which suggest that certain structures cause mental health problems (id, ego, superego, core beliefs, lack of internal locus of control, etc.). Rather than harbor on past problems that tend to be embedded in oppressive belief systems, post-modern approaches suggest that clients can find exceptions to their problems and develop creative solutions. Post-modern approaches tend to be short-term therapies, with solution-focused brief therapy being considered a particularly brief approach, sometimes lasting fewer than five sessions.

APPENDIX E

CLINICAL CASE REPORT

1. Demographic Information
Name:_____ D.O.B.:_____
Address:_____ Age:_____
Phone:_____ Sex:_____
E-Mail:_____ Ethnicity:_____
Name of Interviewer:_____ Date of Interview:_____

2. Presenting Problem or Reason for Referral
1. Who referred the client to the agency?
2. What is the main reason the client contacted the agency?
3. Reason for assessment?

3. Family Background
1. Significant factors from family of origin
2. Significant factors from current family
3. Some specific issues that may be mentioned: where the individual grew up, sex and ages of siblings, whether the client came from an intact family, who were the major caretakers, important stories from childhood, sex and age of current children, significant others, and marital concerns

4. Significant Medical/Counseling History
1. Significant medical history, particularly anything that may affect issues related to the client's assessment (e.g., emotional status for a therapeutic assessment, physical status for an assessment of disability)
2. Types and dates of previous counseling

5. Substance Use and Abuse
1. Use or abuse of food, cigarettes, alcohol, prescription medication, and illegal drugs
2. Counseling related to use and abuse

6. Educational and Vocational History
1. Educational history (e.g., level of education and possibly names of institutions)
2. Vocational history and career path (names and types of jobs)
3. Satisfaction with educational level and career path
5. Significant leisure activities

7. Other Pertinent Information
1. Legal concerns and history of problems with the law
2. Issues related to sexuality (e.g., sexual orientation, sexual dysfunction)
3. Financial problems
4. Other?

8. The Mental Status Exam
1. Appearance and behavior (e.g., dress, hygiene, posture, tics, non-verbals, manner of speech)
2. Emotional state (e.g., affect and mood)
3. Thought components (e.g., content and process: delusions, distortions of body image, hallucinations, obsessions, suicidal or homicidal ideation, circumstantially, coherence, flight of ideas, logical thinking, intact as opposed to loose associations, organization, and tangentiality)
4. Cognitive functioning (e.g., oriented to time, place, and person; short- and long-term memory; knowledge base and intellectual functioning; insight and judgments)

9. Assessment Results
1. List of assessment and test instruments used
2. Summary of results
3. Avoid raw scores and state results in unbiased manner
4. Consider using standardized test scores and percentiles

10. Diagnosis
1. DSM-IV-TR diagnoses (other diagnoses, such as medical, rehabilitation, when important)
2. Usually note all five axes of DSM-IV-TR
   Axis I: Clinical Disorders and Other Conditions That May Be a Focus of Clinical Attention
   Axis II: Personality Disorders and Mental Retardation
   Axis III: General Medical Conditions
   Axis IV: Psychosocial and Environmental Problems
   Axis V: Global Assessment of Functioning, or GAF Scale

11. Summary and Conclusions
1. Integration of all previous information
2. Accurate, succinct, and relevant
3. No new information
4. Inferences that are logical, sound, defendable, and based on facts in the report
5. Try to have at least one paragraph that speaks to the client's strengths

12. Recommendations
1. Based on all the information gathered
2. Should make logical sense to reader
3. In paragraph form or as a listing
4. Usually followed by signature of examiner

APPENDIX F

CONSULTATION AT A MENTAL HEALTH CENTER

The Problem

The administrative director of a small mental health agency has contacted you because there is infighting among the staff. The outpatient staff does not get along with the day treatment staff, who do not get along with the inpatient staff (see descriptions below). There are some problems, also, with the clerical staff.

The Staff: Directors

Clinical Director

You have a doctorate in clinical psychology, and you are in charge of this agency. You are bright, sharp, and have dedicated your whole life to making sure things run smoothly. You are upset that consultants have been called, because you take this as a personal attack on your style of managing the agency. However, you will try to work with them. You feel as though no one works as hard as you do, and at times, that makes you frustrated with your staff. Because Inpatient Counselor 3 lacks insight and may have molested clients a number of years ago, you would like to see that counselor fired. The administrative director is concerned that Inpatient Counselor 3 will sue the agency if he gets fired and has blocked your attempts to do so. You have no evidence regarding the molestation rumors. You are a licensed psychologist.

Medical Director

You see yourself in charge of the agency and often have turf battles with the Clinical Director. You believe that medication should be used more frequently than it is, and you're frustrated with the staff's lack of knowledge about psychopharmacology. You had an affair with Counselor 1, but that is now behind you. You make a lot of money. You are a board-certified psychiatrist.

Administrative Director

You are generally concerned about the functioning of the agency and the relationships of your staff. However, you are also concerned about the money being brought into the agency and that insurance companies are not always billed correctly. You are concerned about retention and follow-up of clients. You would like to see fewer clients receiving a "sliding scale" and attract more clients who have insurance. You have an MBA. You believe everyone at the agency should have or be working on their license.

Director of Consultation and Education

You have a doctorate in counseling and have been hired to run or sponsor workshops for the community. You periodically see clients in the outpatient unit, but generally you are in the community doing PR for the agency. You like the agency, and you are hopeful about its future expansion. You seem happy, but secretly you are quite depressed and at times suicidal.

You are 44, never married, and lonely. Your job is your life. You are not licensed. Despite the fact that you are on paper a "director," you have no staff under you. This creates an identity problem for you at the agency.

The Staff: The Outpatient Staff

Outpatient Counselor 1

You have a master's degree in counseling. You have been working in this agency for 15 years and are an experienced counselor, but sometimes you act a little too much like "the expert." You are married and had an affair with the Medical Director. The affair ended, and you feel a little bitter about the whole event. You are an LPC. You secretly believe that Outpatient Counselor 2 obtained his (or her) job because of his (her) race—the agency needed to hire a minority to better match the makeup of clients in the community. Despite the fact that the outpatient staff has some internal problems, when it comes down to it, you get along with one another. With the exception of the outpatient staff, you see the rest of the agency as "the enemy."

Outpatient Counselor 2

You have a master's degree in social work and are new to the agency and fresh out of school. You are single and "looking" and can't wait until work's over to get out to the local "scene." You say you want to learn, but act as though you know everything already. You think the agency is a little uptight. You are African American, and you think that others treat you as being a little "special" because of that fact. You don't like Outpatient Counselor 5's strict adherence to a family therapy modality. Despite the fact that the outpatient staff has some internal problems, when it comes down to it, you all get along with one another. With the exception of the outpatient staff, you see the rest of the agency as "the enemy."

Outpatient Counselor 3

You have a doctorate in counseling psychology and have worked at the agency for five years. You're looking for another job. You tend not to like anyone at the agency and generally have a negative attitude. You are married and have four children. You and your spouse are expecting again. You really are sick and tired of Outpatient Counselor 4's happy attitude all the time, and you don't like Outpatient Counselor 5's strict adherence to a family therapy modality. You are working on becoming licensed. Despite the fact that the outpatient staff has some internal problems, in tough times, you stick together. With the exception of the outpatient staff, you see the rest of the agency as "the enemy."

Outpatient Counselor 4

You have a master's degree in human resources. There is a push to get everyone licensed in the agency, and you would have to go back to school to pick up additional course work in counseling to be eligible to be licensed. You don't want to do this, but you know it's inevitable.

You are always happy. You like everyone and everything you do. You wish that everyone would be happy and get along like a family. If they could, then you could reveal to them, like you revealed to your own family, the fact that you are gay (or lesbian). Instead, you harbor this secret. Despite the fact that the outpatient staff has some internal problems, when it comes down to it, you get along with one another. With the exception of the outpatient staff, you see the rest of the agency as "the enemy."

Outpatient Therapist 5/School Counselor

You have a master's degree in school counseling, have taken a number of courses in family therapy, and are working toward your LPC. You are hired half-time at the agency and half-time at a local school system. The agency pays your benefits, and you see yourself more as a mental health counselor than as a school counselor. You consult with that school system and end up seeing, at the agency, some of the more "difficult" students.

You see yourself as a family therapy specialist, and at times the staff thinks you go overboard with seeing families rather than individuals. You resent this and believe you know the right way to work with clients. You are a bit of a social isolate at the agency because you are not there half of the time. You know about the affair of Outpatient Counselor 1 with the Medical Director and believe it is a sign that the agency is dysfunctional. Despite the fact that the outpatient staff has some internal problems, when it comes down to it, you get along with one another. With the exception of the outpatient staff, you see the rest of the agency as "the enemy."

The Staff: Inpatient Staff

Inpatient Counselor 1

You have the same degree as the outpatient counselors but get treated as a second-class citizen within the agency. You make less money than the outpatient therapists, and you are bitter about this. You actually feel inferior clinically but don't want the staff to know this.

You have been out of school one year. Despite the fact that the inpatient staff has some internal problems, when it comes down to it, you get along with one another. With the exception of the inpatient staff, you see the rest of the agency as "the enemy."

Inpatient Counselor 2

You have a bachelor's degree in human services. You are directive in your counseling style, and the staff has been trying to tone you down a little. They are concerned that you don't have the skills to work with clients who have severe pathology. You see this job as temporary before going back for your master's degree. You are young but don't realize it. Despite the fact that the inpatient staff has some internal problems, when it comes down to it, you get along with one another. With the exception of the inpatient staff, you see the rest of the agency as "the enemy."

Inpatient Counselor 3

You have worked in the agency for 20 years. Rumor has it that a number of years ago, you molested one of the patients. You seem friendly, but most of the staff does not like to get too close to you because of the rumors. You are married and have a family. You seem to lack insight into your own behavior. You have a master's degree in social work, and you're not licensed. Despite the fact that the inpatient staff has some internal problems, when it comes down to it, you get along with one another. With the exception of the inpatient staff, you see the rest of the agency as "the enemy."

The Staff: Day Treatment Specialists

Day Treatment Specialist 1

You have worked at the agency for 12 years with the chronically mentally ill. You are burnt out, cynical, and at times even hostile. You believe your salary is abysmally low. You also don't like the fact that the day treatment program is seen as the worst job in the agency. You have a brother who recently died of AIDS, and you are quite depressed about this. No one in the agency knows this, but it is clearly affecting your work. You have a bachelor's degree in psychology.

Despite the fact that the day treatment staff has some internal problems, when it comes down to it, in tough times, the three of you will support one another. With the exception of the day treatment staff, you see the rest of the agency as "the enemy."

Day Treatment Specialist 2

You are very good friends with Day Treatment Specialist 3. Both of you dislike Day Treatment Specialist 1. You are young and enthusiastic. You chose to enter this field because you have a sister who is chronically schizophrenic, and you thought you could help people with similar problems. You are beginning work on your master's degree in counseling along with Day Treatment Specialist 3. You are a little arrogant. Despite the fact that the day treatment staff has some internal problems, when it comes down to it, in tough times the three of you will support one another. With the exception of the day treatment staff, you see the rest of the agency as "the enemy."

Day Treatment Specialist 3

You are very good friends with Day Treatment Specialist 2. Both of you dislike Day Treatment Specialist 1. You are young and enthusiastic. You are beginning work on your master's degree in counseling along with Day Treatment Specialist 2. You view the patients as being sick. You have an incredible crush on Secretary 2 to the point where you spend a lot of time during work hours with her. Despite the fact that the day treatment staff has some internal problems, when it comes down to it, in tough times the three of you will support one another. With the exception of the day treatment staff, you see the rest of the agency as "the enemy."

The Staff: Clerical Staff

Program Specialist 1 (Secretary 1)

You have worked at the agency for 20 years, and you are the "surrogate parent" of the agency. The staff always see you as a motherly figure. You know about everyone's life, and sometimes people think you really run the agency.

Program Specialist 2 (Secretary 2)

You just finished secretarial school, and you're happy to have this job. Although you state and believe that you take confidentiality seriously, the truth of the matter is that you tell your friends about the clients. You're 19 years old, very attractive, and go out with various people at the agency from time to time.

APPENDIX G

UNDERSTANDING YOUR HOLLAND CODE

After discovering which of the Holland codes most represents your personality type, you can find out which corresponding job environments best match you. For instance, a person with an investigative personality would want to find investigative jobs (e.g., scientist, mathematician).

A brief description of each of the personality types and some jobs that fit that type can be found at the end of this appendix. Examine the descriptions and the sample jobs to see if they seem to fit the way you see yourself. Keep in mind that no description will perfectly fit any person. In reviewing each description, most likely it would benefit you to try to find a job that fits both your personality type and its corresponding work environment.

Often, it is important to find a job that not only matches your highest personality type but has qualities of your second and third orientation also. For instance, an individual who has a fairly high social and artistic orientation might be interested in jobs like counselor, teacher, physical therapist, minister, and so on, because all of these jobs have both a social and artistic component to them.

Holland did research that supported the notion that the six personality types could be viewed on a hexagon (see below), with those that are next to one another being similar and those on opposite sides being different from one another.

Probably, in discovering your personality codes, you have found that they are adjacent on the hexagon. This would make sense because the orientations adjacent to one another share more in common than do the types that are opposite. Similarly, most jobs do not exclusively follow one personality type but also offer some of the qualities of the orientation closest on the hexagon. If, however, you found that your highest personality types are not adjacent to one another, it is likely that you will have fewer job settings from which to choose. In some cases, this will make your job search more difficult.

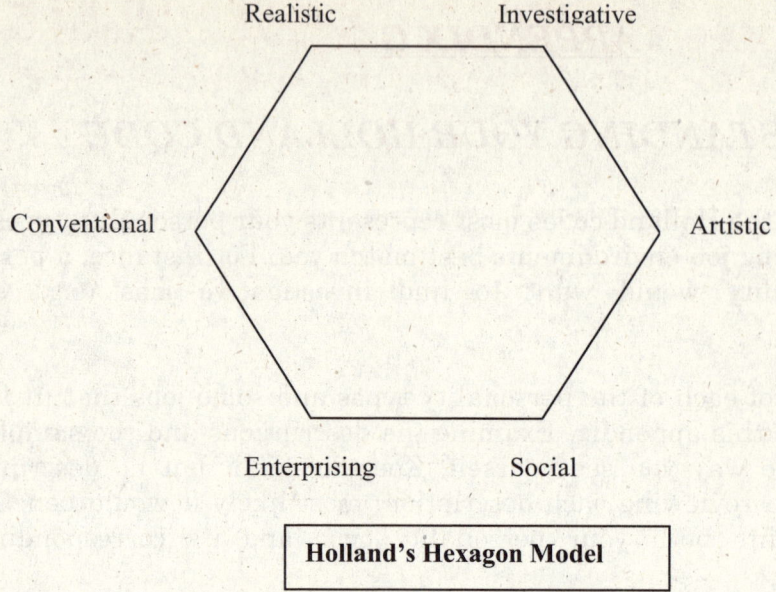

Holland's Hexagon Model

Keep in mind that there are approximately 30,000 jobs in this country, and, at this point, we are offering you only a small sample of the kinds of jobs that might fit your personality type. If you would like to examine other related jobs after taking the inventory, there are a number of things you can do. First, you can go to a career counselor who, using a number of sophisticated instruments, can further the identification of your Holland personality type. Secondly, you can go online and visit the *Dictionary of Occupational Titles* (DOT), which offers descriptions of nearly 13,000 jobs (see http://www.occupationalinfo.org/). This important resource, published by the U.S. Employment Service, offers a listing of all jobs in the United States, which you can cross-reference with your personality type. In addition, since the DOT is being phased out in preference for a database called O*NET, you can visit this online site and obtain descriptions of over 1,000 commonly held jobs (see http://online.onetcenter.org/). Finally, you can simply go online and search for "Holland Codes." I think you will be surprised by the amount of information you will find.

THE CODES

REALISTIC: Realistic people like to work with equipment, machines, or tools, often prefer to work outdoors, and are good with manipulating concrete physical objects. These individuals prefer to avoid social situations, artistic endeavors, or intellectual tasks. They are often practical, robust, and have good physical skills. Realistic people tend to do well in work environments that promote the use of large motor skills and athletic and/or technical skills, and places where they do not have to take on leadership roles.

Some settings in which you might find realistic individuals include filling stations, farms, machine shops, construction sites, and power plants. Some typical jobs include forester, locksmith, animal trainer, farmer, machinist, geologist, mechanical engineer, cook, bricklayer, electrician, plumber, automobile or airplane mechanic, draftsperson, machine operator, and/or surveyor.

INVESTIGATIVE: Investigative people like to think abstractly, problem solve, and investigate. These individuals feel comfortable with the pursuit of knowledge and the manipulation of ideas and symbols. They prefer scientific methodology and feel comfortable with foreign languages, reading, arithmetic, and the arts. Investigative individuals prefer to avoid social situations and see themselves as introverted. They tend to do well in work environments that promote independence, originality, and scholarly pursuits.

Some settings in which you might find investigative individuals include research laboratories, hospitals, universities, and government-sponsored research agencies. Some typical jobs include microbiologist, biologist, dentist, physician, chemist, scientist, physicist, research psychologist, geneticist, biochemist, civil engineer, assistant to scientist, dietitian, veterinarian, nurse practitioner, geologist, researcher, mathematician, computer programmer, and/or laboratory technician.

ARTISTIC: Artistic individuals like to express themselves creatively, usually through artistic forms such as drama, art, music, and writing. They prefer unstructured activities in which they can use their imagination and creative side. They tend to prefer work environments that allow them to express their independence, sensitivity, and emotional side. They crave originality and flexibility at the workplace.

Some settings in which you might find artistic individuals include the theater, concert halls, libraries, art or music studios, dance studios, orchestras, photography studios, newspapers, and restaurants. Some typical jobs include comedian, actor, dancer, musician, conductor, designer, artist, writer, photographer, drama and art teacher, pastry chef, editor, sculptor, and/or music teacher.

SOCIAL: Social people are nurturers, helpers, and caregivers, and have a high concern for others. They are introspective and insightful and prefer work environments in which they can use their intuitive and care-giving skills. They tend to be responsible citizens and usually have good communication skills. They prefer work settings where there is much social interaction and where they can use their social and helping skills.

Some settings in which you might find social people are government social service agencies, counseling offices, churches, schools, mental hospitals, reaction centers, personnel offices, and hospitals. Some typical jobs include counselor, psychologist, minister, speech therapist, social worker, psychiatric aid, social science teacher, chiropractor, nurse supervisor, human service worker, political scientist, nurse, sociologist, teacher, college professor, and/or educational administrator.

ENTERPRISING: Enterprising individuals are self-confident, adventurous, bold, and sociable. They have good persuasive skills and prefer positions of leadership. They tend to dominate conversations and enjoy work environments in which they can satisfy their need for recognition, power, and expression. They tend to be good public speakers and appear emotionally stable.

Some settings in which you might find enterprising individuals include life insurance agencies, advertising agencies, political offices, real estate offices, new and used car lots, sales offices, and in management settings. Some typical jobs include life insurance agent, realtor, politician, broker, hotel clerk, sales, manager, business executive, sales manager, manager of personnel, car salesperson, and/or jobs in which there is a need for management, supervision, or administration of programs.

CONVENTIONAL: Individuals of the conventional orientation are stable, controlled, conservative, and sociable. They prefer working on concrete tasks and like to follow instructions. They like routine problem-solving and working with data. They would prefer a work environment that is orderly and neat, and in which their tasks are clear and spelled out. They value the business world and clerical tasks and tend to be good at computational skills.

Some settings in which you might find conventional people include banks, business offices, accounting firms, and medical records. Some typical jobs include data entry clerk, bookkeeper, accountant, stenographer, machine duplicator, receptionist, secretary, teller, banker, tax expert, credit manager, payroll clerk, file clerk, and/or a variety of other clerical positions.

Reproduced by special permission of the Publisher, Psychological Assessment Resources, Inc., 16204 North Florida Avenue, Lutz, FL 33549, from *Making Vocational Choices*, 3rd ed., Copyright 1973, 1985, 1992, 1997 by Psychological Assessment Resources, Inc. All rights reserved.

APPENDIX H

THE NORMAL CURVE WITH TYPES OF STANDARDS SCORES

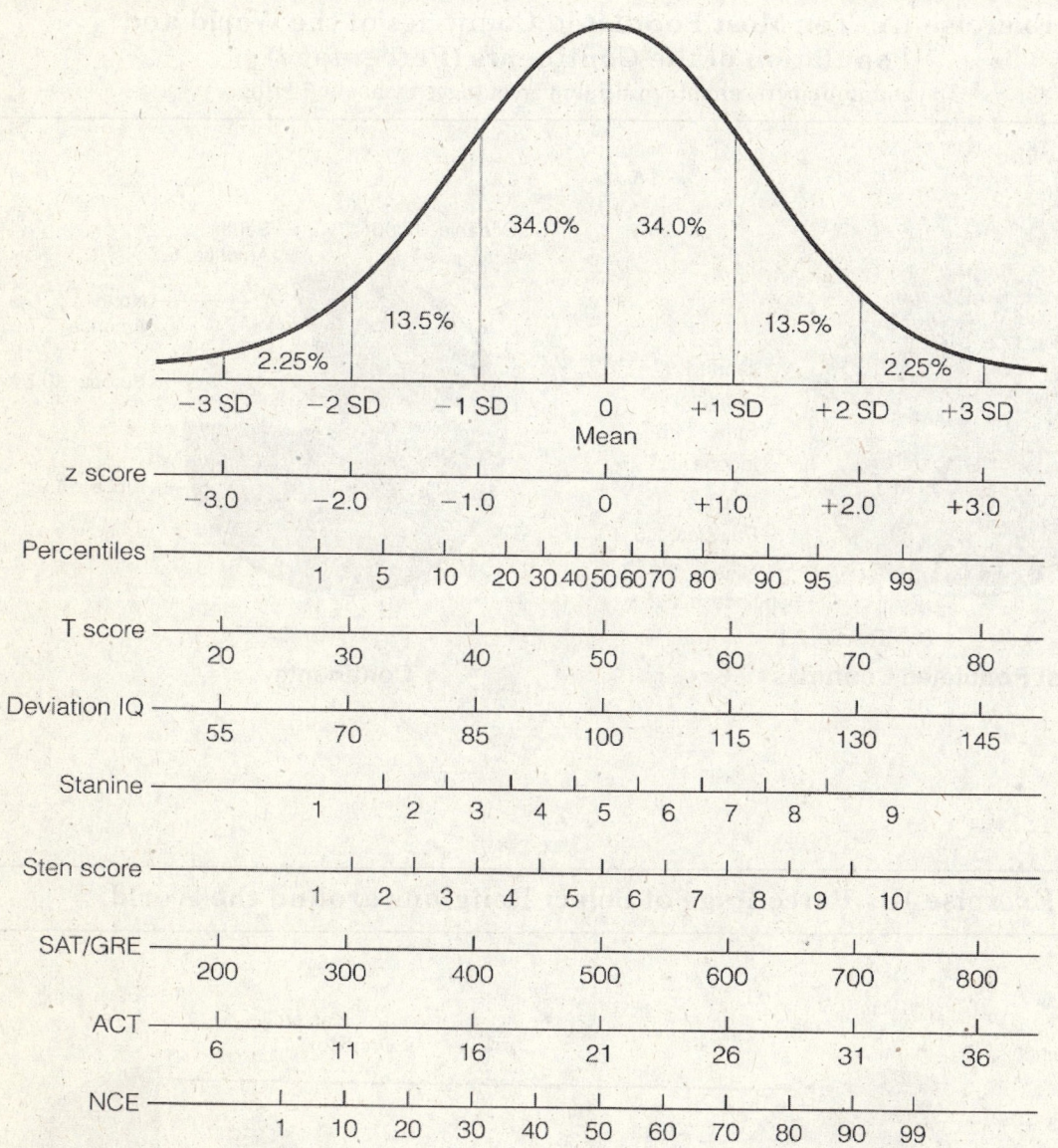

203

APPENDIX I

NUMBERS AND PERCENTAGES OF PEOPLE AND RELIGIONS IN THE WORLD*

> **Exercise 1A: Ten Most Populated Countries of the World and Population of the Continents (Percentage)**
> To obtain numbers, simply multiply percentages by about 7 billion.

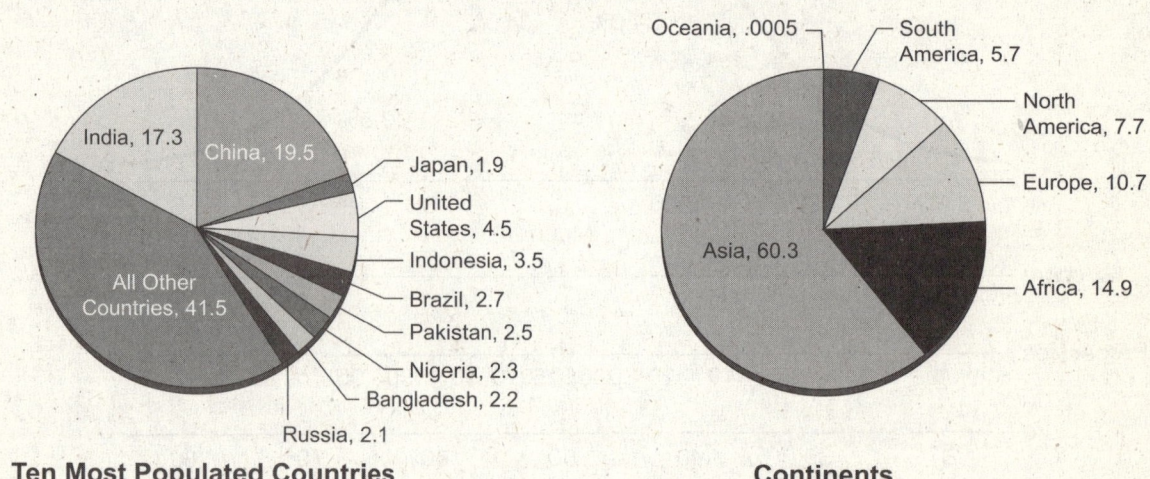

Ten Most Populated Countries

- China, 19.5
- India, 17.3
- Japan, 1.9
- United States, 4.5
- Indonesia, 3.5
- Brazil, 2.7
- Pakistan, 2.5
- Nigeria, 2.3
- Bangladesh, 2.2
- Russia, 2.1
- All Other Countries, 41.5

Continents

- Oceania, .0005
- South America, 5.7
- North America, 7.7
- Europe, 10.7
- Africa, 14.9
- Asia, 60.3

> **Exercise 1B: Percentage of Select Religions around the World**

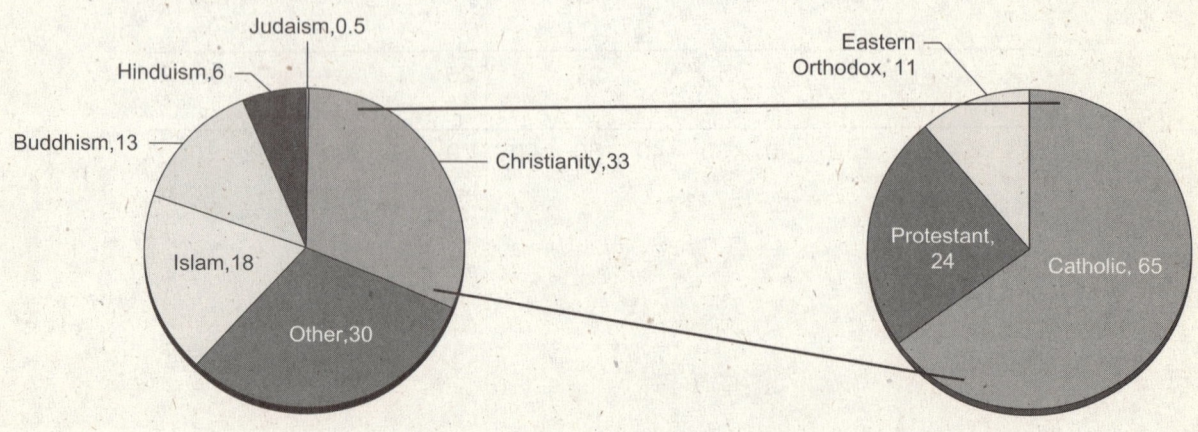

- Judaism, 0.5
- Hinduism, 6
- Buddhism, 13
- Islam, 18
- Other, 30
- Christianity, 33
  - Eastern Orthodox, 11
  - Protestant, 24
  - Catholic, 65

Exercise 1.C: Number and Percentage of Individuals from Select Racial, Ethnic, Cultural, Religious, and Sexual Identity Backgrounds in the United States

ETHNICITY/RACE*	Number (In Millions)	Percentage
White	199.8	65.1
Hispanic	48.4	15.8
Black or African American	41.8	13.6
Asian	16.0	4.3
American Indian and Alaska Native (AIAN)	5.0	1.6
Native Hawaiian and other Pacific Islander (NHPI)	1.1	<1
Two or More Races	5.4	1.7

SEXUAL ORIENTATION**		
Gay		2.5
Lesbian		1.4
Gay, Lesbian, or Bisexual		4.1

Religion***	Number (In Millions)	Percentage
Christian	173	76.0
Christian (non-Catholic)	116	50.9
Catholic	57	25.1
Select Religious and Nonreligious Groups		
Baptist	36	15.8
Christian Generic	32	14.2
Mainline Christians (Methodist, Lutheran, Episcopalian, United Church of Christ)	29	12.9
Pentecostal	7.9	3.5
Mormon	3.2	1.4
Jewish	2.7	1.2
Eastern Religions (e.g., Buddhist)	2.0	.9
Muslim	1.3	.6
Atheist/Agnostic	3.5	1.6
None	34	15.0

Figures from United States Census Bureau (2009). Hispanics are treated as one group, and they identify as 92% Caucasian, 4% African American, 1.6% AIAN, 1.5% two races, .6% Asian, and .3% NHPI. Group members may identify with more than one race. Thus, the groups add up to more than the total population of the United States. Caucasians listed are non-Hispanic. Caucasian with Caucasian Hispanic equals 84% of the population.

** Gay and lesbian figures are based on a narrow definition of individuals who have engaged exclusively in same-sex sex over one year (Black, Gates, Sanders, & Taylor, 2000). Gay, lesbian, or bisexual figures are difficult to assess (Center for Disease Control, 2002).

***From Kosmin, B. A., & Keysar, A. (2008). Number of Jews is based on religious identification and is a smaller number than those who identify as Jewish. The number of Muslims is probably much higher, as many mosques do not officially affiliate as a religious denomination.

APPENDIX J

GRADUATE DEGREE EXPLORATION WORKSHEET

Is graduate study for you? If the answer is yes, then how do you find the program that fits you best? This worksheet will assist you in making this decision and help you find the programs that are right for you. As you complete this worksheet, you will not only identify graduate programs that are a good fit, but you will also be creating a road map that you can follow to help increase your chances of being accepted into a graduate program.

Step 1: Goal Clarification

The best way to know if graduate study is right for you is to know what you want to do and have at least a rough idea of your ambitions. *Identify four or five professional/vocational goals based on your personal desires and aspirations, keeping in mind your desired income and lifestyle. Examine your motives, willingness, and determination to continue for the two to seven more years that it will take to obtain a masters and/or doctoral degree.*

1. _____

2. _____

3. _____

4. _____

5. _____

Step 2: Degree Exploration

Two levels of graduate degrees are conferred in human services: master's and doctoral degrees. To help meet your professional/vocational goals, you need to be familiar with both. Master's degree preparation (M.S., M.A., M.Ed.) is typically the entry-level requirement for clinical practice in professional counseling, social work, and marriage and family therapy. Psychology (Ph.D., Psy.D., Ed.D.) and psychiatry (M.D., D.O.) require doctoral-level preparation for entry-level practice. You need to know what each of the curriculums emphasizes to make the most informed decision. *Identify two master's degree and two doctoral degree programs that interest you from the resources identified in Chapter 15, Section IV: Finding a Graduate School. List the commonalities of both types of programs including mission, curriculum, qualifications of graduates, etc.*

Master's Degree Programs						Commonalities

_____			_____

_____			_____

Doctoral Degree Programs					Commonalities

_____			_____

_____			_____

Step 3: Recognize Resources

The realities of the application process and costs associated with graduate study can be considerable. Application costs include the required exams, transcripts, application fees, postage, and expenditures related to the interview process. Once accepted, the costs for tuition, fees, books and other expenses add up quickly. Recognizing your financial limitations relating to the application process can help prepare you to be fiscally responsible for paying for graduate school once admitted. You need to consider the costs and inquire about funding opportunities, including scholarships, assistantships, work study opportunities, program/campus-related employment, and flexibility of course work to accommodate employment outside of school (see Step 8, Personal Contact). *Create a budget based on your current financial resources that will result in the maximum amount you can commit to the application process (refer to Chapter 15, Section III: Applying to Graduate School). Then create a two-to-three-year proposed budget based on your current and immediate future financial obligations, i.e., car payments, living expenses, debts, etc.).*

Step 4: Program Identification

Identifying the right graduate programs for you to apply to is imperative. There are several factors to consider when making this decision. Based on the goals you identified in Step 2 and the type of degree you desire from Step 3, review the resources identified in Chapter 15, Section IV: Finding a Graduate School. Identify five to eight programs that seem to match your responses and record the following information related to the admissions criteria and pertinent program information.

Step 5: Program Categorization
Categorize the programs you identified in Step 4 into two groups (refer to the resources identified in Chapter 15, Section IV: Finding a Graduate School). The first group includes programs that you feel confident about gaining access to based on qualifications and program requirements; the second group also matches you well but its requirements are more stringent than your qualifications. This two-fold approach will allow you to select programs that match who you are, your needs, and resources. Things to consider: admissions criteria and new student acceptance rates.

Prospective Programs Group 1
1. _____
2. _____
3. _____
4. _____

Prospective Programs Group 2
1. _____
2. _____
3. _____
4. _____

Step 6: Prepare Credentials
The strongest applicants set themselves apart from other applicants, so prepare your undergraduate experience accordingly and seek out broad opportunities. Things to consider include involvement in honor societies such as PSI CHI; involvement in clubs and leadership opportunities; seeking out research opportunities with undergraduate faculty; seeking out opportunities to attend professional conferences and training outside (professional organizations such as the ACA and APA market and promote conferences/workshops); and interviewing and getting to know professionals in the community that have attained the type of credentials and career you are seeking.

Step 7: Application Process
Know and meet the application requirements. Create a timetable for all tasks to be done. Creativity is the name of the game so that your materials stand apart while still remaining within the application's guidelines. Thoroughness is crucial. Become a perfectionist with applications, essays, and writing samples. Have your application materials reviewed by one of your undergraduate professors familiar with the type of program(s) for which you are applying.

Step 8: Personal Contact
Applying does not end when you submit your application materials. Keep in contact with the program throughout the application process and ask questions. Get to know the names of the department secretary and the faculty who teach in the program. It is advisable that you make initial contact with program representatives prior to submitting the application to ask questions related to Step 4, Program Identification. The strongest applicants are not solely known to prospective programs by virtue of the application materials but also by their demonstrated interest and engagement in the application process through personal contact.

*Adapted from McCurdy, K. G. (1998, July). Should you get your Ph.D.? *Counseling Today*. Alexandria, VA: American Counseling Association. A special thanks to Dr. Ken McCurdy, Gannon University, for forwarding this contribution to us.